Manual on

PREVENTIVE ONCOLOGY

AF729917

Manual on PREVENTIVE ONCOLOGY

Series Editors

Nandita Palshetkar
MD FCPS FICOG FRCOG (UK)
Professor Emeritus
Department of Obstetrics and Gynecology
DY Patil School of Medicine, Navi Mumbai,
Maharashtra, India
Founder and Medical Director of the
Famous Bloom IVF Group

Hrishikesh D Pai
MD FRCOG (UK-HON) FCPS FICOG MSc (USA)
Trustee, FIGO, Asia Oceania (2023–25)
Professor, DY Patil University, Navi Mumbai,
Maharashtra, India
Immediate Past President FOGSI (2022–23)
Founder and Medical Director, Bloom IVF
Group, Mumbai

Niranjan Chavan
MD FICOG FCPS DGO DFP MICOG DICOG Diploma in Endoscopy (USA)
Professor and Unit Chief
Department of Obstetrics and Gynecology
Lokmanya Tilak Medical College and General Hospital
Mumbai, Maharashtra, India

Editors

Priya Ganesh Kumar
MBBS MD DGO DFP FICOG
Medical Director of Sainiwas
Healthcare, Pan India
Chairperson Gynaecologic Oncology
Committee FOGSI 2021–24
WHO/IARC/FOGSI Colposcopy
Course Trainer
Master Trainer for Cervical Cancer
Prevention Under NCD for State Govt. MP
Convenor of FOGSI GCPR on Cervical
Cancer Prevention and Management 2023

Charulata Bapaye
MBBS MD
Chief Mentor and Director
GEMS Hospital and Endoscopy Centre
Pune, Maharashtra, India
Consultant at Deenanath Mangeshkar
Hospital, Oyster and Pearl Hospital and
Jahangir Hospital, Pune
Past Visiting Professor at the Department of
Physiotherapy, Fergusson College, Pune
Past Organizing Secretary
International Conferences
"Pearls and Pitfalls in
Gynec Endoscopy and ART"

Girish Mane
MBBS DGO MD(USAIM) FICOG MBA (Hospital Management)
Director and Senior Consultant, Mane Hospital
Yavatmal, Maharashtra, India
State Coordinator, Maharashtra Obstetrics and Gynaecological Societies

Co-Editors

**Helen Kamei, Alpesh Gandhi, Neeraj Bhatla,
Amrita Tandon, Ashwini Kalyankar, Pramod Survase**

JAYPEE

JAYPEE BROTHERS MEDICAL PUBLISHERS
The Health Sciences Publisher
New Delhi | London

Message from Series Editors

Dear AICOG 2025 delegates,

It is a matter of great pride that the landmark AICOG 2025 is being held in the city of Mumbai, Maharashtra, India. The Organizing Committee and the hosts Mumbai Obstetric and Gynaecological Society have left no stone unturned in their quest to make this a historic event by aiming to have a scientific program of the highest caliber, punctuated by fantastic keynotes and orations, graced by the best international faculty in the field of Obstetrics, Gynecology and its subspecialities along with a cultural treat every evening to cater to the audience which hails from far-flung corners of India and the globe.

On this occasion, the academic stalwarts and senior FOGSIans have burned the midnight oil at both ends to contribute and create a set of AICOG 2025 Workshop Manuals that aim to amalgamate the most recent scientific advancements and evidence-based best practices in a nutshell for the delegates to take home and implement in their practices when they have returned from this magnificent event.

We acknowledge the efforts of all the editors, co-editors, authors, co-authors, co-contributors and junior authors who have sometimes worked at short notice to submit excellent chapters and articles included in the final publication. We also wish to take this opportunity to thank Shri Jitendar P Vij (Group Chairman) and Mr Ankit Vij (Managing Director) of M/s Jaypee Brothers Medical Publishers (P) Ltd, New Delhi, India, in publishing the book and their associates, particularly Ms Chetna Malhotra (Senior Director—Professional Publishing, Marketing, and Business Development), Ms Kritika Dua (Senior Commissiong Editor), and Mr Priyansh Saxena (Development Editor), who have been prompt, efficient, and most helpful.

We hope that the delegates and the attendees will enjoy reading this publication and the scientific data included therein will help to shape your knowledge, attitudes and practices and ultimately benefit the women of our country, whom we all serve.

Nandita Palshetkar
Organizing Chairperson, AICOG Mumbai, 2025

Hrishikesh D Pai
Chairperson, Scientific Committee, AICOG Mumbai, 2025

Niranjan Chavan
Organizing Secretary, AICOG Mumbai, 2025

Jaypee Brothers Medical Publishers (P) Ltd

Headquarters
Jaypee Brothers Medical Publishers (P) Ltd
EMCA House, 23/23-B
Ansari Road, Daryaganj
New Delhi 110 002, India
Landline: +91-11-23272143, +91-11-23272703
+91-11-23282021, +91-11-23245672
Email: jaypee@jaypeebrothers.com

Corporate Office
Jaypee Brothers Medical Publishers (P) Ltd
4838/24, Ansari Road, Daryaganj
New Delhi 110 002, India
Phone: +91-11-43574357
Fax: +91-11-43574314
Email: jaypee@jaypeebrothers.com

Overseas Office
JP Medical Ltd.
83, Victoria Street, London
SW1H 0HW (UK)
Phone: +44 20 3170 8910
Fax: +44 (0)20 3008 6180
Email: info@jpmedpub.com

Website: www.jaypeebrothers.com
Website: www.jaypeedigital.com

Inquiries for bulk sales may be solicited at: jaypee@jaypeebrothers.com

Manual on Preventive Oncology

First Edition: **2025**

ISBN: 978-93-6616-174-7

Printed at: Samrat Offset Pvt. Ltd.

Contributors

Amita Maheshwari
MBBS MS MCH
Professor and Head
Department of Gynecologic Oncology
Tata Memorial Hospital
Mumbai, Maharashtra, India

Anil E
MBBS MD
Consultant (Obstetrics & Gynecology)
Department of Telemedicine
Post Graduate Institute of Medical Education and Research (PGIMER)
Chandigarh, India

Anju Singh
MBBS MD
Associate Professor
Department of Obstetrics and Gynecology
All India Institute of Medical Sciences
New Delhi, India

Bhagyalaxmi Nayak
PhD
Professor
Department of Gynecologic Oncology
Acharya Harihar Post Graduate Institute of Cancer
Cuttack, Odisha, India

Bindiya Gupta
MBBS MD MAMS FICOG
Professor
Department of Obstetrics and Gynecology
UCMS and GTB Hospital
New Delhi, India

Chiranjeev Shetty
MBBS
Junior Resident
Department of Obstetrics and Gynecology
DY Patil School of Medicine
Navi Mumbai, Maharashtra, India

Devika Kamat
MBBS MD
MCh Fellow
Gynecologic Oncology
All India Institute of Medical Sciences
Rishikesh, Uttarakhand, India

Geetha Balsarkar
MBBS MD DGO DNB FCPS
Editor-in-Chief
Professor and Unit Head
Nowrosjee Wadia Maternity Hospital
Mumbai, Maharashtra, India

Harshad Parasnis
MD DNB FCPS DGO FICOG FICS
Consultant Gynecologic Oncologist,
President, Pune Obst-Gyn Soc, 2020–2021
Head of Gynec Oncology Unit and Associate Professor
Bharati Medical College, Pune
Hon Gynecologic Oncologist BJGMC and Sassoon General Hospital, Pune
Chairperson, Oncology Committee, FOGSI (2009–2011)
Chairperson, Oncology Committee, AMOGS (2020–2022)

Helen Kamei
MBBS MS (Obs & Gyne) Fellowship in Gynecologic Oncology
Professor
Gyne-Oncology Unit
Department of Obstetrics and Gynecology
JNIMS
Manipur, India

Kanmani Murugesan
MBBS MCH
Senior Resident
Department of Gynecologic Oncology
Tata Memorial Hospital
Mumbai, Maharashtra, India

Karishma Kirti
MBBS MS
Surgeon
Palshetkar Patil Nursing Home
Mumbai, Maharashtra, India

Kirti Shankhdhar
MBBS DNB DGO
Director
Dr Kirti's Women's Health Clinic
Mumbai, Maharashtra, India

Mala Srivastava
MBBS DNB DGO
Professor GRIPMER and Senior Consultant Institute of Obstetrics and Gynecology
Sir Ganga Ram Hospital
New Delhi, India

Mayanglambam Ronita Devi
MBBS MS (Obs & Gyne) FICOG
Colposcopy Trainee
Assistant Professor
Department of Obstetrics and Gynecology
JNIMS
Imphal, Manipur, India

Mayuri More
MBBS MS (Obs & Gyne) FRM (ICOG) DRM (Germany)
Consultant
DY Patil Fertility Centre (Bloom IVF), Navi Mumbai
Assistant Professor
DY Patil School of Medicine
Navi Mumbai, Maharashtra, India

Meenal Bhati
MBBS MS
Senior Resident
MCh Gyne Oncology
Department of Obstetrics and Gynecology
All India Institute of Medical Sciences
New Delhi, India

Monika Dewan
MBBS MD
Consultant
Department of Gynecologic Oncology
SSIMS
Gwalior, Madhya Pradesh, India

Nandita Palshetkar
MD FCPS FICOG FRCOG (UK)
Professor Emeritus
Department of Obstetrics and Gynecology
DY Patil School of Medicine
Navi Mumbai, Maharashtra, India
Founder and Medical Director of the Famous Bloom IVF Group

Neerja Bhatla
MBBS MD FICOG MAMS
Ex-Professor and HOD
Department of Obstetrics and Gynecology
All India Institute of Medical Sciences
New Delhi, India

Niranjan Chavan
MD FICOG FCPS DGO DFP MICOG DICOG Diploma in Endoscopy (USA)
Professor and Unit Chief
Department of Obstetrics and Gynecology
Lokmanya Tilak Medical College and General Hospital
Mumbai, Maharashtra, India

Nita S Nair
MBBS MCh MRCS
Consultant
Breast Oncosurgeon
Apollo Hospital
Mumbai, Maharashtra, India

Priya Ganesh Kumar
MBBS MD DGO DFP FICOG
Medical Director of Sainiwas Healthcare, Pan India
Chairperson Gynaecologic Oncology Committee FOGSI 2021–24

WHO/IARC/FOGSI Colposcopy Course Trainer
Master Trainer for Cervical Cancer Prevention Under NCD for State Govt. MP
Convenor of FOGSI GCPR on Cervical Cancer Prevention and Management 2023

Rashmi Bagga
MBBS MD
Professor
Department of Obstetrics and Gynecology
Post Graduate Institute of Medical Education and Research (PGIMER)
Chandigarh, India

Rohan Palshetkar
MS (Obs & Gyne) FRM BDRME ADRME
Professor at DY Patil Medical College
Unit Head of DY Patil Bloom IVF and Opera House Bloom IVF
Chairperson of the FOGSI Young Talent Promotion Committee

Ruchi Chokshi
MBBS DNB MRCOG FCPS DGO BSCCP (Colposcopist)
Senior Clinical Fellow (Office Gynecology, Colposcopy and High-Risk Obstetrics) Obstetrician and Gynecologist
Great Western Hospital
Swindon, UK

Saloni Chadha
MBBS MS (MAMC) DrNB
Gynecologist and Oncologist
Safdarjung Hospital and VMMC
New Delhi, India

Samar Gupte
MBBS MD
Gynecologic Oncologist
Hinduja Hospital, Surya Hospital, Wadia Hospital, Gupte Clinic and Breach Candy Hospital
Mumbai, Maharashtra, India

Sarita Bhalerao
MBBS MD DNB FCPS DFP FRCOG
Diploma in Pelvic Endoscopy
Consultant Obstetrician and Gynecologist
Bhatia, Saifee, Reliance HNH, Breach Candy Hospitals
Mumbai, Maharashtra, India
Secretary ICOG

Seema Singhal
MBBS MS MCh (Gyn Oncology) FACS FCLS
Gynecologic Oncologist, Additional Professor
Department of Obstetrics and Gynecology
All India Institute of Medical Sciences
New Delhi, India

Shalini Rajaram
MBBS MD
Professor and Program Lead
MCh Gynecologic Oncology
All India Institute of Medical Sciences
Rishikesh, Uttarakhand, India

Sholanki Haldar
MBBS MS
Senior Resident
MCh Gyne Oncology
Department of Obstetrics and Gynecology
All India Institute of Medical Sciences
New Delhi, India

Usha Saraiya
MD DGO FIAC FICOG FRCOG
Visiting Oncologist, Cama and Albless Hospital and Consultant Obstetrician and Gynecologist at Breach Candy Hospital and Research Centre and Saifee Hospital
Mumbai, Maharashtra, India

Preface

Preventive Oncology as a subject has been evolving and continues to be, with advances in understanding regarding risk factors, etiopathogenesis, better and advanced diagnostic modalities and a leap changes in treatment, which focuses more on cure and quality of life. However, our country diversity in terms of health care facilities and infrastructure have been a major hurdles in terms of delivery of health care services. The cervical malignancy associated morbidity data and mortality data are still dismal, especially considering the World Health Organization declaration for the elimination of cervical cancer.

An early diagnosis or better yet, effective prevention measure can be affected only if there is a good understanding of how to approach and evaluate a case with chance of or established gynecological malignancy. This workshop manual has been brought forth with the sole purpose of helping a busy, practicing gynecologist and postgraduate trainees to effect a proper approach and evaluation for proper diagnosis and timely treatment.

We acknowledge the dedication of the authors for their contribution and the staffs involved with the publication. We hope the manual will serve the sole purpose intended, which is improving the health care for patients with gynecological malignancy

Series Editors: Nandita Palshetkar, Hrishikesh D Pai, Niranjan Chavan
Editors: Priya Ganesh Kumar, Charulata Bapaye, Girish Mane
Co-Editors: Helen Kamei, Alpesh Gandhi, Neeraj Bhatla, Amrita Tandon, Ashwini Kalyankar, Pramod Survase

Contents

Section 1 Introduction to Gynecological Malignancies

1. **Gynecological Malignancies Overview** 3
Helen Kamei, Priya Ganesh Kumar, Mayanglambam Ronita Devi

Section 2 Naughty Silent Ovarian Cancer

2. **Pathophysiology of Ovarian Cancer** 9
Ruchi Chokshi, Sarita Bhalerao

3. **Screening in Ovarian Cancer** 15
Bindiya Gupta

4. **Diagnosis and Treatment of Ovarian Cancer from a Gynecologist's Perspective** 20
Shalini Rajaram, Devika Kamat

5. **Persistent Unruptured Ovarian Cyst: How to Proceed?** 28
Rashmi Bagga, Anil E

Section 3 Endometrial Cancer: Red Flag

6. **New FIGO Classification of Endometrial Cancer** 39
Seema Singhal, Meenal Bhati, Sholanki Haldar

7. **Screening for Endometrial Cancer** 52
Geetha Balsarkar

8. **Lynch Syndrome** 56
Mala Srivastava, Saloni Chadha

9. **Radical Hysterectomy: The Wertheim's Surgery** 62
Samar Gupte

Section 4 Cervical Cancer: Prevent the Preventable

10. **Pathophysiology of Cervical Cancer with FIGO Staging** 69
Anju Singh, Neerja Bhatla

11. **FOGSI-GCPR for Cervical Cancer Prevention and Management** 74
Priya Ganesh Kumar

12. **Adenocarcinoma of Cervix: An Emerging Issue** 82
Usha Saraiya

13. **Radical Trachelectomy** 90
Harshad Parasnis

Section 5 Vulvar and Vaginal Carcinoma: Untouched Domain

14. **Basics of Vulvar Anatomy with Benign and Malignant Vulvar Diseases** 97
Niranjan Chavan, Helen Kamei

15. **Various Treatment Modalities of Vulva and Vaginal Diseases** 104
Bhagyalaxmi Nayak, Monika Dewan

16. **Surgery for Vulvar Cancer** 110
Kanmani Murugesan, Amita Maheshwari

Section 6 Miscellaneous

17. **Breast Cancer Screening** 127
Karishma Kirti, Nita S Nair

18. **Colposcopy Manual** 135
Priya Ganesh Kumar, Kirti Shankhdhar

19. **Fertility Preservation in Gynecological Cancer** 146
Rohan Palshetkar, Nandita Palshetkar, Mayuri More, Chiranjeev Shetty

1

SECTION

Introduction to Gynecological Malignancies

1. **Gynecological Malignancies Overview**
   Helen Kamei, Priya Ganesh Kumar, Mayanglambam Ronita Devi

1

CHAPTER

Gynecological Malignancies Overview

Helen Kamei, Priya Ganesh Kumar, Mayanglambam Ronita Devi

The burden of cancers globally is increasing and globally, gynecological cancers are the most common cancer among women. GLOBOCAN 2020 noted that amongst gynecological cancers—breast, cervical, ovarian, and uterine cancers ranked amongst the top 10 common cancers in women globally.[1] Breast cancer has been found to be one of the most common cancers among women worldwide; on the other hand, in some developing countries, cervical cancer remained a leading cause of cancer-related deaths.[2,3] From 1990 to 2021, data [the Global Burden of Disease (GBD) Study, 2021] covering 204 countries and territories were analyzed on the incidence and disability-adjusted life years (DALYs) of four major female cancers (breast, cervical, uterine, and ovarian cancer) among 15–49 years women.[4] An estimate of 1,013,475 new female cancers cases were reported globally in 2021. Between 1990 to 2021, the increase in age-standardized incidence rate (ASIR) (estimated annual percentage changes, EAPC 0.16%) with a decrease in age-standardized DALYs rate (–0.73%) were found to be significant. Except for cervical cancer, an annually increasing trends of age-standardized incidence rate were observed for the remaining cancers. Breast and cervical cancers were prevalent worldwide, compared to ovarian and uterine cancers. The age-standardized incidence rates of breast, ovarian, and uterine cancers showed an increasing trend along with increasing sociodemographic index (SDI). On the other hand, cervical cancer had downward trends for both ASIR and DALY rates along with SDI. The increase of age-specific rates of female cancers with age in 2021 was significantly notable in younger age groups, except for uterine cancer.[4] Variations in incidence and mortality have been noted geographically too. A population-based study was carried out for the epidemiological trends of women's cancers based on data from GBD spanning 1990 to 2019;[5] for breast cancers, the USA, China, and Germany were the top three countries with the most incidence cases in 1990; by 2019, China (368.37×10^3), the USA (251.53×10^3), and India (144.09×10^3) were the countries with the most incidence cases, China (93.50×10^3), India (82.10×10^3), and the USA (54.40×10^3) were the countries with the most deaths. Worldwide cervical cancer has been in decreasing trends since past three decades. However, high SDI countries had the lowest incidence and mortality rate while low SDI countries had highest incidence and mortality rate in 2019. The highest cancer burden was in middle SDI countries. China, India, and Brazil were leading countries for cervical cancer incidence and mortality. The highest burden of ovarian cancer and mortality fell on high SDI countries; low SDI despite lower burden and mortality, it had the most rapid increase in ASIR and mortality. The uterine cancer incidence increased in 2019, but the mortality rate has decreased during the past three decades. The incidence and mortality were highest in high SDI countries with the USA, China, and Russia as the leading countries in terms of incidence, with India ranking sixth in 2019.[5] Cancer of vulva and vagina are less common among the gynecological malignancies, but cause as much morbidity and mortality.

Much advancements have been seen in terms of diagnosis, disease understanding and treatment, be it surgery, radiation, or chemotherapy; thus, bringing about better cure rates, improvement in quality of life, progression free survival and overall survival. Understanding of the natural history of cervical cancer starting with the Human Papilloma Virus, has made the possibility of achieving "cervical cancer eradication" a reality to be seen soon. Another reality about gynecological cancer is that in low-middle income countries, cancer of the breast, cervix, ovary, uterus, vagina, and vulva still account for nearly one-fourths deaths of overall cancer.[6] The key to reducing any cancer incidence, mortality, and morbidity would be preventive measures, modifiable lifestyle risk factors and early detection with effective treatment strategies. Unlike cervical cancer, even though much needs to be done before achieving the goal of eradication, other gynecological malignancies do not have effective screening and primary preventive strategies. GLOBOCAN 2022 reported 1,437,427 new gynecological cancer cases with almost half of the figure related to mortality—680,372 deaths. An analysis of global burden of gynecological cancers in 2022 with projections to 2050 reverberate about the global disparities in incidence and mortality and concluded that the number of gynecological cancer cases in the next two decades will rise if the current trends continue and highlighted about the needs for interventions that can effectively prevent it.[7] The objective of the following chapters is to bring about better understanding of the basics of gynecological malignancies in terms of organ-specific cancer for practicing gynecologists, to affect an intervention that would help bring down the overall incidence and mortality related to gynecological malignancies.

REFERENCES

1. Sung H, Ferlay J, Siegel RL, Laversanne M, Soerjomataram I, Jemal A, et al. Global Cancer Statistics 2020: GLOBOCAN estimates of incidence and mortality worldwide for 36 cancers in 185 countries. CA Cancer J Clin. 2021;71:209-49.

2. Li N, Deng Y, Zhou L, et al. Global burden of breast cancer and attributable risk factors in 195 countries and territories, from 1990 to 2017: results from the global burden of disease study 2017. J Hematol Oncol. 2019;12(1):140.
3. Canfell K, Kim JJ, Brisson M, et al. Mortality impact of achieving WHO cervical cancer elimination targets: a comparative modelling analysis in 78 low-income and lower-middle-income countries. Lancet. 2020;395(10224):591-603.
4. Sun P, Yu C, Yin L, Chen Y, Sun Z, Zhang T, et al. Global, regional, and national burden of female cancers in women of child-bearing age, 1990–2021: analysis of data from the global burden of disease study 2021. EClinicalMedicine. 2024;74:102713.
5. Yi M, Li T, Niu M, et al. Epidemiological trends of women's cancers from 1990 to 2019 at the global, regional, and national levels: a population-based study. Biomark Res. 2021;9(1):55.
6. International Association for Research on Cancer. Cancer today. Geneva: World Health Organization. https://gco.iarc.fr/today/home.
7. Zhu B, Gu H, Mao Z, Beeraka NM, Zhao X, Anand MP, et al. Global Burden of Gynaecological Cancers in 2022 and Projections to 2050. J Glob Health. 2024;14:04155.

SECTION 2

Naughty Silent Ovarian Cancer

2. **Pathophysiology of Ovarian Cancer**
   Ruchi Chokshi, Sarita Bhalerao
3. **Screening in Ovarian Cancer**
   Bindiya Gupta
4. **Diagnosis and Treatment of Ovarian Cancer from a Gynecologist's Perspective**
   Shalini Rajaram, Devika Kamat
5. **Persistent Unruptured Ovarian Cyst: How to Proceed?**
   Rashmi Bagga, Anil E

2 CHAPTER

Pathophysiology of Ovarian Cancer

Ruchi Chokshi, Sarita Bhalerao

INTRODUCTION

Ovarian cancer is a complex and often devastating malignancy that poses significant challenges for gynecologists in India. As the third most common cancer among Indian women, with an age-adjusted incidence rate of 6.8 per 100,000,[1,2] it demands a thorough understanding of its pathophysiology for effective management and improved patient outcomes.

TYPES OF OVARIAN CANCER

Epithelial Ovarian Cancer

Epithelial ovarian cancer (EOC) accounts for approximately 90% of all ovarian malignancies. It is further classified into several subtypes of which serous is the most common subtype.

High-grade serous carcinoma (HGSC)[3] is the most common and aggressive form, representing about 70% of EOCs. The peak age range is 45–65 years. HGSCs are characterized by rapid growth, early metastasis, and poor prognosis. High-grade serous epithelial ovarian carcinoma, fallopian tube and peritoneal carcinomas are considered a single clinical entity due to their shared clinical behavior and treatment. They typically exhibit p53 or BRCA1/2 mutations and genomic instability.

Low-grade serous carcinoma (LGSC) is less common <5% and is typically diagnosed at an advanced stage, and consequently the long-term prognosis is poor. LGSCs often harbor KRAS or BRAF mutations and are associated with a more indolent clinical course.[4]

Endometrioid carcinoma accounts for about 10% of EOCs and is frequently associated with endometriosis. It is also associated with carcinoma of the endometrium in 15–20% of cases. These tumors often exhibit mutations in *PTEN* and *ARID1A* genes.[5]

Mucinous carcinoma represents 3–4% of EOCs and is characterized by mucin-producing cells. Approximately, 80% are benign mucinous cystadenomas and majority of borderline neoplasms. These tumors often have KRAS mutations and may be associated with pseudomyxoma peritonei.[6]

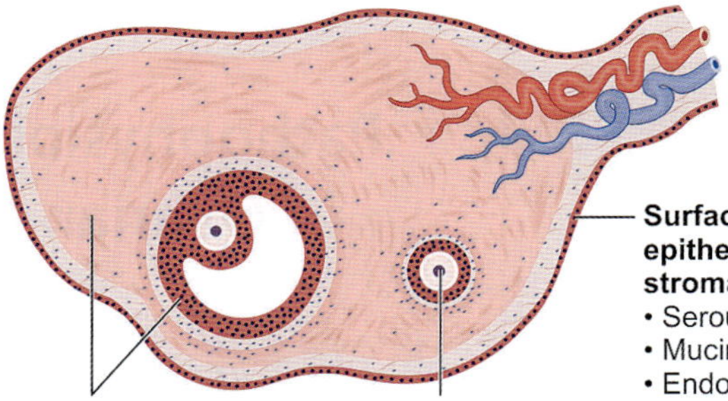

Fig. 1: Epithelial and nonepithelial types—ovarian cancer.

Clear cell carcinoma comprises about 5–10% of EOCs and is also associated with endometriosis. Tubal ligation has been shown to be protective against the development of ovarian clear cell carcinoma. These tumors frequently harbor *KRAS, PTEN, PIK3CA,* and *ARID1A* mutations and have a distinct molecular profile.[7]

Nonepithelial Types[8]

Germ cell tumors arise from primordial germ cells and account for about 3% of ovarian cancers. They are more common in younger women and include subtypes such as dysgerminomas and yolk sac tumors.

Stromal tumors originate from the sex cord-stromal cells of the ovary and represent about 7% of ovarian cancers. These include granulosa cell tumors and Sertoli-Leydig cell tumors **(Fig. 1)**.

BORDERLINE NEOPLASMS

These group of neoplasms typically lack obvious malignant characteristics but sometimes exhibit intraperitoneal spread.[9] They represent 14–15% of all primary ovarian tumors. Initially, the "borderline" category was applied only to serous neoplasms, but it has since been recognized that mucinous, endometrioid, and clear cell neoplasms also fall within this category.

PATHOPHYSIOLOGIC MECHANISMS

Genetic Mutations and Pathways[10]

The pathogenesis of ovarian cancer involves multiple genetic alterations and molecular pathways. Key mutations include:

- *TP53:* Nearly ubiquitous in HGSC, contributing to genomic instability and aggressive behavior.

- *BRCA1/2:* Germline mutations in these genes significantly increase the risk of ovarian cancer, particularly HGSC.
- *KRAS and BRAF:* Common in LGSC and mucinous carcinomas, affecting cell proliferation and survival.

The two-pathway hypothesis proposes distinct mechanisms for ovarian carcinogenesis:[11]

1. *Type I tumors (LGSC, endometrioid, clear cell, and mucinous carcinomas)* develop in a stepwise manner from precursor lesions and are characterized by specific mutations (e.g., KRAS, BRAF, PTEN).
2. *Type II tumors (primarily HGSC)* develop rapidly without well-defined precursor lesions and are characterized by TP53 mutations and chromosomal instability.

Cellular Origins and Transformation

The cellular origin of ovarian cancer has been a subject of debate.[12] Traditional views suggested that ovarian surface epithelium (OSE) and cortical inclusion cysts were the primary sources of EOC. However, recent evidence supports the fallopian tube epithelium, particularly the fimbriated end, as the origin of many HGSCs.

The transformation process involves:

- Accumulation of genetic mutations
- Loss of cell cycle control
- Evasion of apoptosis
- Acquisition of invasive properties

TUMOR DISSEMINATION PATTERNS

Lymphatic Spread

Ovarian cancer commonly spreads through lymphatic channels. The primary lymphatic drainage routes include:

- Para-aortic lymph nodes
- Pelvic lymph nodes (external iliac, internal iliac, and obturator)

Understanding these patterns is crucial for accurate staging and surgical planning.

Metastasis

Peritoneal spread is the most common form of metastasis in ovarian cancer. Malignant cells can detach from the primary tumor and implant on peritoneal surfaces, leading to widespread abdominal disease. Hematogenous spread, while less common, can result in distant metastases to organs such as the liver and lungs.

HISTOLOGICAL AND MOLECULAR CLASSIFICATION

Histological Subtypes

HGSC, the most common subtype, is characterized by:

- Marked nuclear atypia
- High mitotic index
- Solid growth pattern with slit-like spaces
- Frequent areas of necrosis

Other subtypes have distinct histological features that aid in diagnosis and classification.

Immunohistochemical Markers

Immunohistochemistry plays a crucial role in diagnosis and classification. Key markers include:[13]

- WT-1 and p53 for HGSC
- PAX8 for Müllerian origin
- Napsin A, Hypoxia-inducible factor 1 alpha (HIF-1 alpha) and hepatocyte nuclear factor 1-beta (HNF-1 beta) for clear cell carcinoma.

These markers help differentiate ovarian cancer subtypes and distinguish primary ovarian tumors from metastases.

CLINICAL IMPLICATIONS FOR GYNECOLOGISTS

Diagnosis and Staging

Understanding the pathophysiology of ovarian cancer is essential for accurate diagnosis and staging.[14] Gynecologists should:

- Recognize the diverse histological subtypes and their clinical behavior
- Utilize appropriate imaging and biomarker tests
- Perform comprehensive surgical staging when indicated

Risk Factors and Prevention

Identifying high-risk individuals is crucial for prevention and early detection. Key risk factors include:[15]

- *Genetic predisposition:* BRCA1/2 mutations confer a lifetime risk of 39–44% and 11–17% for ovarian cancer, respectively.
- *Family history:* First-degree relatives with ovarian cancer increase risk.
- *Age:* Risk increases with age, peaking in the late 60s and 70s.

Gynecologists should consider genetic counseling and testing for appropriate patients and discuss risk-reducing strategies, such as prophylactic salpingo-oophorectomy for high-risk individuals.

CONCLUSION

The pathophysiology of ovarian cancer is complex and multifaceted, involving various genetic, molecular, and cellular processes. Understanding these mechanisms is crucial for gynecologists to provide optimal care for patients in India. As research continues to unravel the intricacies of ovarian cancer pathogenesis, new opportunities for targeted therapies and improved diagnostic approaches are emerging.

Future directions in ovarian cancer research include:
- Identifying novel biomarkers for early detection
- Developing targeted therapies based on molecular profiles
- Exploring immunotherapeutic approaches
- Investigating strategies to overcome chemoresistance.

By staying informed about the latest developments in ovarian cancer pathophysiology, gynecologists can contribute to improved patient outcomes and advance the field of gynecologic oncology in India.

REFERENCES

1. Webb PM, Jordan SJ. Global epidemiology of epithelial ovarian cancer. Nat Rev Clin Oncol. 2024;21(5):389-400. doi: 10.1038/s41571-024-00881-3. Epub 2024 Mar 28. PMID: 38548868.
2. Meena RK, Syed NA, Sheikh ZA, et al. Patterns of Treatment and Outcomes in Epithelial Ovarian Cancer: A Retrospective North Indian Single-Institution Experience. JCO Glob Oncol. 2022;8:e2200032. doi: 10.1200/GO.22.00032. PMID: 36332174; PMCID: PMC9668559.
3. Bowtell DD, Böhm S, Ahmed AA, et al. Rethinking ovarian cancer II: reducing mortality from high-grade serous ovarian cancer. Nat Rev Cancer. 2015;15(11):668-79. doi: 10.1038/nrc4019. PMID: 26493647; PMCID: PMC4892184.
4. Slomovitz B, Gourley C, Carey MS, et al. Low-grade serous ovarian cancer: State of the science. Gynecol Oncol. 2020;156(3):715-25. doi: 10.1016/j.ygyno.2019.12.033. Epub 2020 Jan 20. PMID: 31969252.
5. Pecorino B, Laganà AS, Chiantera V, et al. Progression Free Survival, Overall Survival, and Relapse Rate in Endometrioid Ovarian Cancer and Synchronous Endometrial-Ovarian Endometrioid Cancer (SEO-EC): Results from a Large Retrospective Analysis. Medicina (Kaunas). 2022;58(12):1706. doi: 10.3390/medicina58121706. PMID: 36556908; PMCID: PMC9784653.
6. Gershenson DM, Okamoto A, Ray-Coquard I. Management of Rare Ovarian Cancer Histologies. J Clin Oncol. 2019;37(27):2406-15. doi: 10.1200/JCO.18.02419. Epub 2019 Aug 12. PMID: 31403866.
7. Gil-Martin M, Pardo B, Barretina-Ginesta MP. Rare ovarian tumours. Other treatments for ovarian cancer. EJC Suppl. 2020;15:96-103. doi: 10.1016/j.ejcsup.2019.11.002. PMID: 33240448; PMCID: PMC7573466.
8. Cheung A, Shah S, Parker J, Soor P, Limbu A, Sheriff M, Boussios S. Non-Epithelial Ovarian Cancers: How Much Do We Really Know? Int J Environ Res

Public Health. 2022;19(3):1106. doi: 10.3390/ijerph19031106. PMID: 35162125; PMCID: PMC8834485.

9. Colombo N, Sessa C, du Bois A, et al; ESMO-ESGO Ovarian Cancer Consensus Conference Working Group. ESMO-ESGO consensus conference recommendations on ovarian cancer: pathology and molecular biology, early and advanced stages, borderline tumours and recurrent disease†. Ann Oncol. 2019;30(5):672-705. doi: 10.1093/annonc/mdz062. PMID: 31046081.
10. Lheureux S, Gourley C, Vergote I, Oza AM. Epithelial ovarian cancer. Lancet. 2019;393(10177):1240-53. doi: 10.1016/S0140-6736(18)32552-2. PMID: 30910306.
11. Tossetta G, Inversetti A. Ovarian Cancer: Advances in Pathophysiology and Therapies. Int J Mol Sci. 2023;24(10):8930. doi: 10.3390/ijms24108930. PMID: 37240277; PMCID: PMC10219114.
12. Kroeger PT Jr, Drapkin R. Pathogenesis and heterogeneity of ovarian cancer. Curr Opin Obstet Gynecol. 2017;29(1):26-34. doi: 10.1097/GCO.0000000000000340. PMID: 27898521; PMCID: PMC5201412.
13. Kim YN, Chung YS, Lee JH, et al. Application of precision medicine based on next-generation sequencing and immunohistochemistry in ovarian cancer: a real-world experience. J Gynecol Oncol. 2023;34(6):e70. doi: 10.3802/jgo.2023.34.e70. Epub 2023 Jun 26. PMID: 37417298; PMCID: PMC10627761.
14. O'Shea AS. Clinical Staging of Ovarian Cancer. Methods Mol Biol. 2022;2424:3-10. doi: 10.1007/978-1-0716-1956-8_1. PMID: 34918284.
15. Berek JS, Renz M, Kehoe S, et al. Cancer of the ovary, fallopian tube, and peritoneum: 2021 update. Int J Gynaecol Obstet. 2021;155 Suppl 1 (Suppl 1):61-85. doi: 10.1002/ijgo.13878. PMID: 34669199; PMCID: PMC9298325.

CHAPTER 3

Screening in Ovarian Cancer

Bindiya Gupta

INTRODUCTION

Ovarian cancer is 7th most common cancer in women worldwide and most lethal amongst all gynecological cancers. It is the 5th most common cause of cancer related death among women.[1] According to the GLOBOCAN 2020, incidence age standardized rate (ASR) and mortality ASR of ovarian cancer worldwide were 6.6 and 4.2 per 100,000 women respectively.[1] There were 239,000 new cases and 152,000 deaths due to ovarian cancer worldwide annually in 2020.[1] Incidence differs in different age and race groups, and is higher in less developed countries. In India, ASR incidence and mortality of ovarian cancer in 2018 was 4.9 and 3.6 per 100,000 women respectively[1] and in 2020 ASR incidence of ovarian cancer was 6.4 per 100,000 women according to NCRP–ICMR, 2020.

Due to lack of screening techniques, nonspecific symptoms in early disease and failure of early detection, ovarian cancer presents in advanced stages. Approximately 70% of patients are present in advanced stage due to delayed onset of symptoms and lack of proper screening tools. Overall, 5-year relative survival rate ranges between 30 and 40% across the globe and has seen only very modest increase (2–4%) since 1995.[2] Early-stage ovarian cancers have a survival rate of 90% versus 30–40% in advanced stages.[3]

Factors which predispose to ovarian cancer include infertility (based on the incessant ovulation theory and the gonadotropin theory), family history/genetic factors (*BRCA1, BRCA2* gene mutations or *MSH2, MLH1, PMS1,* and *PMS2* gene mutations in Lynch II syndrome) and previous hormone therapy.[4] Other factors responsible for increase in incidence are decrease pregnancy rate, lack of lactation, cigarette smoking, alcohol consumption, use of talc, obesity (BMI >25) and other high-risk factors such as polycystic ovary syndrome, pelvic inflammatory disease, endometriosis, etc.

SCREENING METHODS

- *Goff symptom index:* It consists of symptoms including bloating, increase abdominal size, feeling full, difficulty eating, loss of appetite, pelvic or abdominal pain, urinary urgency or frequency and weight loss. If the symptoms are persistent (>12 times a month) in less than 1 year, the sensitivity was 56.7% for early-stage disease; 79.5% for advanced-stage disease and specificity was 90% for women age >50 years.[5]

- *Pelvic examination:* There is insufficient evidence to assess the balance of benefits and harms of performing screening pelvic examinations in asymptomatic, nonpregnant adult women for detection of ovarian cancer.
- *Tumor marker:* Serial CA125 has a positive predictive value of 40% for detecting invasive ovarian cancer. It is elevated in 50% of stage 1 disease and 90% in stages 2–4. It may be also elevated in fibroids, endometriosis, menstruation and tuberculosis, and other cancers (breast, bladder, liver, lungs, pancreas).
- *Transvaginal sonography (TVS):* Measuring the ovarian volume and ovarian morphology on transvaginal sonography is a useful adjunct to CA125. The main limitations are that aggressive tumors metastasize before reaching sonographically detected size, subjective nature of assessment and interobserver variations, difficult visualization of ovaries (obese, hysterectomized, tubal ligated) and poor visualization of fallopian tubes and tumor <1 cm. Newer techniques are been developed to improve accuracy including Doppler flow parameters, microbubble contrast-enhanced ultrasonography, photoacoustic imaging and advanced imaging techniques like use of immunological biomarkers such as modified macrophages targeting cancer cells and nanoprobes.

GUIDELINES FOR SCREENING IN AVERAGE RISK WOMEN[10]

The US Preventive Services Task Force (USPSTF) recommends against screening for ovarian cancer in asymptomatic women (Grade D recommendation). Ovarian cancer mortality did not differ between screened women and those with no screening or in usual care. Screening harms included surgery (with major surgical complications) in women found to not have cancer.

GUIDELINES FOR SCREENING IN HIGH-RISK WOMEN (HEREDITARY CANCER RISK)[11]

Genetic counseling and testing should be offered to both affected and unaffected women with increased likelihood for the disease. Individuals with significant family history should be offered genetic testing using multigene panels of clinically validated *HBOC* genes but clinicians should be aware that family history-based testing misses about half of HBOC syndrome gene carriers, and strategies to identify these high-risk individuals are being developed.

Pretest genetic counseling: A detailed pedigree analysis and risk assessment should be done to determine eligibility for genetic testing and informed consent should be obtained.

Genetic tests offered include *BRCA1* and *BRCA2* mutations testing or multigene panel testing which includes the intermediate risk genes apart from *BRCA1* and *BRCA2*. Ideally the index case (proband) should be tested. *Post-test counseling* includes reporting and interpretation of the results and discussion of management options.

Women with completed family: The most effective strategy for ovarian cancer risk reduction in BRCA1/2 PV carriers is risk reducing bilateral salpingo-oophorectomy (RRBSO) at 35–40 years of age (BRCA1 carriers) and 40–45 years of age (BRCA2) mutation carriers. RRBSO should be considered in women who have completed childbearing who are carriers of pathogenic variants (PVs) in BRIP1, RAD51C, or RAD51D at age 45–50. RRBSO may be considered for postmenopausal women with a PALB2 PV. Hysterectomy with bilateral salpingo-oophorectomy should be done in Lynch syndrome. Risk-reducing salpingectomy (bilateral salpingectomy alone or bilateral salpingectomy followed by delayed oophorectomy) is not recommended outside the setting of a clinical trial **(Tables 1 and 2)**.

TABLE 1: Trials in general population.

Trials	*Screening strategy*	*Key outcomes*
Prostate, Lung, Colorectal and Ovarian (PLCO)[6] Cancer Screening Trial	CA125 + TVS 4 years Followed by CA125 alone for 2 years	No reduction in mortality (RR 1.06; 95% CI 0.87–1.3)
UK Collaborative Trial of Ovarian Cancer Screening (UKCTOCS)[7]	*Intervention arm:* • *MMS strategy:* Longitudinal CA125 (median 8) (ROCA) followed by TVS and repeat CA125 if risk not in normal range • *USS:* Serial TVS screens strategy (11 annually) *Control arm:* No screening	*At 16.3 years (intervention vs. control arm):* • 1% women diagnosed with ovarian cancer in each group • Compared with no screening, a 47.2% increase in stage 1 and a 25% decrease in stage IV disease incidence in the MMS group • Overall incidence of stage I/II disease was 39.2% higher in the MMS group versus no screening • Incidence of stage III/IV disease was 10.2% lower • 0.6% mortality in the three groups • No significant reduction in ovarian and tubal cancer deaths in MMS ($p = 0.58$) OR USS ($p = 0.36$) groups compared with the no screening group

TABLE 2: Trials in high-risk population.

Trials	*Strategy*	*Key outcomes*
UK Familial Ovarian Cancer Screening Study (UKFOCSS) Phase 1[8]	Annual combined screening of TVS and CA125	• Lacked sensitivity for early-stage disease detection • Improved optimal debulking rates (62%)
UKFOCSS Phase 2[9]	4-monthly CA125 (ROCA) and annual TVS *Eligibility criteria:* >10% lifetime risk of ovarian cancer, age >35 years, declined RRBSO	• Significant increase in low volume disease (Stage I–IIIa vs. IV) • Nonsignificant zero-residual disease after debulking • Significant decrease in use of NACT • *Sensitivity:* 75–100%, specificity of 96.1%, PPV of 13%
US Cancer Genetics Network and Gynecologic Oncology Group trials	3-monthly multimodality screening (CA125)	Significant Increase in stage 1/2 (50% vs. 10% P = 0.01) compared to historical BRCA1 controls

Women desirous of fertility preservation (Short-term surveillance): Screening by TVS 6-monthly and CA125 starting at 30–35 years until definitive risk reduction surgery.

CONCLUSION

Guidelines are in place to recommend risk reduction and screening strategies in high-risk women with inherited risk. Further research is needed to identify effective approaches for reducing ovarian cancer incidence and mortality in general population.

REFERENCES

1. Bray F, Ferlay J, Soerjomataram I, Siegel RL, Torre LA, Jemal A. Global Cancer Statistics 2018: GLOBOCAN estimates of incidence and mortality worldwide for 36 cancers in 185 countries. CA: a Cancer Journal for Clinicians. 2018;68(6):394-424.
2. Reid BM, Permuth JB, Sellers TA. Epidemiology of ovarian cancer: a review. Cancer Biology and Medicine. 2017;14(1):9.
3. Shabir S, Gill PK. Global scenario on ovarian cancer: its dynamics, relative survival, treatment, and epidemiology. Adesh University Journal of Medical Sciences and Research. 2020;2(1):17-25.
4. Patni R. Screening for ovarian cancer: an update. J Midlife Health. 2019;10(1):3-5.
5. Goff BA, Mandel LS, Drescher CW, Urban N, Gough S, Schurman KM, et al. Development of an ovarian cancer symptom index: possibilities for earlier detection. Cancer. 2007;109:221-7.

6. Buys SS, Partridge E, Black A, Johnson CC, Lamerato L, Isaacs C, et al. Effect of Screening on Ovarian Cancer Mortality: the Prostate, Lung, Colorectal and Ovarian (PLCO) Cancer Screening Randomized Controlled Trial. JAMA. 2011;305:2295-303.
7. Menon U, Gentry-Maharaj A, Burnell M, et al. Ovarian cancer population screening and mortality after long-term follow-up in the UK Collaborative Trial of Ovarian Cancer Screening (UKCTOCS): a randomised controlled trial. Lancet. 2021;397(10290):2182-93.
8. Rosenthal AN. Ovarian cancer screening in the high-risk population: the UK Familial Ovarian Cancer Screening Study (UKFOCSS). Int J Gynecol Cancer. 2012;22(Suppl 1):S27-8.
9. Rosenthal AN, Fraser LSM, Philpott S, Manchanda R, Burnell M, et al; United Kingdom Familial Ovarian Cancer Screening Study collaborators. Evidence of Stage Shift in Women Diagnosed with Ovarian Cancer During Phase II of the United Kingdom Familial Ovarian Cancer Screening Study. J Clin Oncol. 2017;35(13):1411-20.
10. US Preventive Services Task Force. Grossman DC, Curry SJ, Owens DK, Barry MJ, Davidson KW, et al. Screening for ovarian cancer: US preventive services task force recommendation statement. JAMA. 2018;319:588-94.
11. Sessa C, et al. Risk reduction and screening of cancer in hereditary breast-ovarian cancer syndromes: ESMO Clinical Practice Guideline· Annals of Oncology. 2022;34(1):33-47.

4 CHAPTER

Diagnosis and Treatment of Ovarian Cancer from a Gynecologist's Perspective

Shalini Rajaram, Devika Kamat

INTRODUCTION

Ovarian cancer is the most lethal gynecological cancer globally. The diagnosis of ovarian malignancy has been a challenge for gynecologists over decades. A screening program for early diagnosis is still not available.[1]

Amongst women who undergo surgical procedures for suspected ovarian neoplasm, 13–21% are found to be ovarian malignancies, thus making it essential to ensure an accurate preoperative diagnosis before treatment. Laparoscopic removal of tumors with suspicion of malignancy has the demerits of inadequate surgical exploration of the peritoneal cavity, risk of spillage, upstaging the disease and instances of port-site metastasis.[2]

Currently, surgical debulking and systemic chemotherapy are typically recommended with or without targeted therapies.[3] Targeted therapy includes antiangiogenic bevacizumab and poly-adenosine diphosphate (ADP)-ribose polymerase (PARP) inhibitors and immunotherapy which have markedly improved survival along with surgical cytoreduction to no visible disease.[4] The majority of cases are diagnosed in advanced stages (III and IV) but the survival rates have improved dramatically.

Ovarian cancer is the seventh most common cancer and sixth leading cause of cancer-related deaths among women worldwide with 3,24,603 new cases and 2,06,956 deaths annually reported in 2022. In India, it the third most common cancer among women with 47,333 new cases and 32978 deaths in 2022.[5] The 5-year relative survival has increased to 50.9% during the 2014–2020 from 47.6% in previous years. 19% of cases are diagnosed when the disease localized to ovaries with a 5-year relative survival rate of 91.9% whereas 55% cases are diagnosed with distant disease and have survival rate of 31.4% (SEER Statistics 2024).[6]

WHO 2020 broadly categorizes ovarian tumors based on different clinicopathological presentation aided by molecular characteristics and immunohistochemical profile. Most of the tumors are categorized as epithelial, mesenchymal, sex cord stromal and germ cell tumors. Immunohistochemistry marker like SALLA4 for germ cell tumors and CD46 and Inhibin for sex cord stromal tumors can be used to distinguish from other subtypes.[7]

Mutations among sex cord stromal tumors are diagnostically significant such as poorly differentiated Sertoli-Leydig cell tumor has DICER1 mutation and adult granulosa cell tumor has mutation in the *FOXL2* gene.[8] Median age at diagnosis of epithelial ovarian cancer is 63 years. While germ cell tumors are predominantly seen in the first to third decades of life, borderline tumors are common in 3rd to 4th decade and invasive epithelial tumors are seen beyond the age of 50 years.[6] The incidence of germ cell tumors is somewhat higher in Asia compared to West.[9]

We now know the origin of high-grade serous carcinomas is from the serous tubal intraepithelial carcinomas (STIC) whereas low-grade serous tumors take their course from benign or borderline serous neoplasms. Endometriosis is found to be associated with clear cell and endometrioid cancers and pelvic inflammatory diseases have dose-response relationship with serous epithelial cancer.[10-12]

Familial ovarian cancers are commonly seen to occur at a younger age. Women with BRCA1 mutation have a lifetime risk of developing ovarian cancer upto 40–50% whereas in BRCA2 mutation the risk is 20–30%.[1] Women with Lynch syndrome carry a risk of endometrial as well as ovarian cancer and should be timely counseled about the need for prophylactic hysterectomy and oophorectomy after completion of family.[10] Lactation, especially longer duration of breastfeeding is associated with decreased risk of epithelial ovarian cancer. Use of oral contraceptives for 5 or more years reduces the risk of developing ovarian cancer to 50%.[10] Prophylatic salpingo-oophorectomy has been proven to reduce the risk among patients with BRCA1 and BRCA2 mutations.[13]

EVALUATION OF AN OVARIAN NEOPLASM

A basic work-up of any adnexal mass should provoke us to diagnose whether a mass is malignant or benign and if symptomatic or not. The adnexal mass may arise from the ovary/fallopian tube/broad ligament/embryological cell rests in the broad ligament. Rarely an appendicular lump, pelvic kidney or colonic mass may present as an adnexal mass. Diagnosis begins with a comprehensive evaluation, including symptoms. Goff's symptom index is a simplified method to assess the symptoms seen in ovarian malignancy. This includes pelvic/abdominal pain, increased abdominal size/bloating, or difficulty eating/feeling full quickly. A woman is positive on the Goff index if she had a new Goff symptom occurring more than 12 times per month within the previous 12 months.[14]

TUMOR MARKERS

CA125 has been the main biomarker used in majority of ovarian cancer. The cut-off value for CA125 is set at 35 U/mL but it may be high in benign conditions, leading to false positives in screening for ovarian cancer. Stage

III–IV endometriosis and genital/abdominal tuberculosis are likely to have raised markedly raised CA125 levels. CA125 is primarily important in the treatment and follow-up phases of ovarian cancer management.[15]

HE4 is a glycoprotein overexpressed in specific ovarian cancer subtypes, with a 100% occurrence in endometroid tumors and 93% in serous histology.[16]

CA19-9 and CEA along with CA125 have been used to differentiate benign, borderline and malignant mucinous ovarian tumors of ovary and are also elevated in gastrointestinal tumors. A CA125 to CEA ratio of >25 is suggestive of an ovarian malignancy.[17]

Inhibin A and B levels are typically undetectable in postmenopausal women and therefore are sensitive markers of sex cord stromal tumors in this population. Inhibin B and anti-Müllerian hormone (AMH) are promising markers for diagnosing and monitoring of granulosa cell tumors especially to detect a recurrence.[16]

Among the germ cell tumors, such as dysgerminomas, LDH may be diagnostic and can also assess treatment response. Placental alkaline phosphatase (PLAP) is utilized as an immunohistochemical marker for dysgerminomas. Typically, pure dysgerminomas are not associated with elevated AFP.

Undifferentiated embryonal carcinomas can synthesize both AFP and HCG. Immature teratomas are derived from embryonic tissues and not associated with raised HCG but may have elevated AFP warranting aggressive treatment.[9]

IMAGING STUDIES

A pelvic ultrasound is the single most effective way of evaluating an ovarian mass with transvaginal ultrasonography being preferable due to its increased sensitivity over transabdominal ultrasound.[18]

RMI (Risk of Malignancy Index) has been commonly used in the risk assessment, taking into consideration the CA125 value, menopausal status (M) and ultrasound characters (U) of the ovarian mass.[19] RMI score <200 is associated with low risk of malignancy. A simple unilocular asymptomatic cyst <5 cm can be managed conservatively with 4–6 monthly follow-up. Such cysts usually resolve over 2–3 menstrual cycles without the need for intervention. RMI score >200 needs further detailed imaging through CT scan and gynecological oncology referral due to higher likelihood of malignancy. This scoring system has also undergone changes such that RMI 1, RMI 2, RMI 3 use the formula of CA125 × M × U and RMI 4 = CA125 × M × U × S (where S stands for size of the lesion: S=1 if size <7 cm and S = 2 if size ≥7 cm).[20]

The International Ovarian Tumour Analysis (IOTA) Group, characterizes the ultrasound findings based on benign features (B rules) and malignant feature (M rules) to have increased sensitivity and specificity. Various models were utilized by the group for preoperative assessment of ovarian masses. The Logistic regression (IOTA LR) model utilizes 12 criteria (for LR1) and six criteria (LR2) for risk assessment of malignancy whereas ADNEX model uses three clinical and six radiological criteria for evaluation.[21]

Ovarian-Adnexal Reporting and Data System Ultrasound (ORADS-US) working group stratified the ovarian masses into six categories based on risk of malignancy: ORADS-US 0—incomplete evaluation; ORADS-US 1—normal premenopausal ovary; ORADS-US 2—the almost certainly benign category (<1% risk of malignancy) **(Fig. 1)**; ORADS-US 3—lesions with low risk of malignancy (1% to <10%); ORADS-US 4—lesions with intermediate risk of malignancy (10% to <50%) **(Fig. 2)**; and ORADS-US 5—lesions with high risk of malignancy (≥50%).[22]

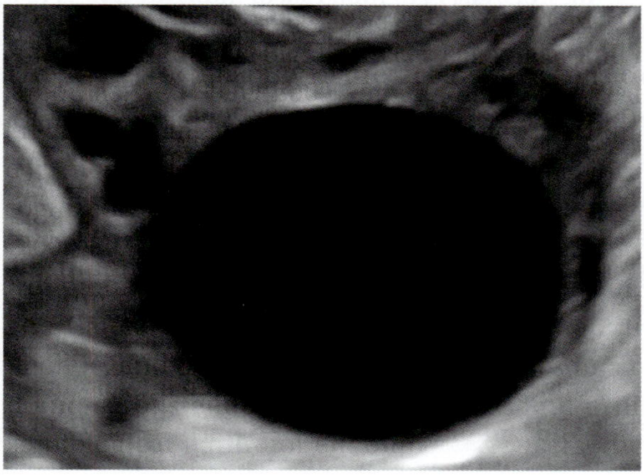

Fig. 1: *ORADS-US 2:* Simple follicular cyst.

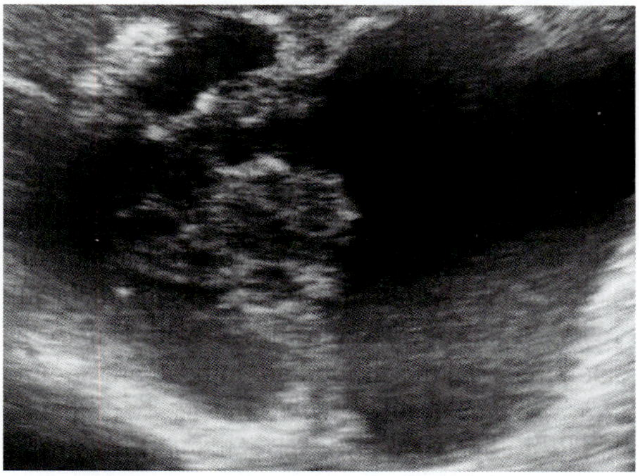

Fig. 2: *ORADS-US 4:* Multilocular cyst with solid appearing component of any size.

A joint consensus statement was released by the European Society of Gynecologic Oncology (ESGO), the International Society of Ultrasound in Obstetrics and Gynecology (ISUOG), the European Society of Gynecologic Endoscopy (ESGE), and IOTA on the use of ORADS-US to determine patient management. According to this consensus, masses classified as ORADS-US 2 should be managed with follow-up, and masses classified as ORADS 3 should be submitted to surgery in general gynecology units. However, masses classified as ORADS-US 4 or 5 should be referred to specialized gynecologic oncology centers.[23]

ORADS-MRI serves to guide risk stratification for adnexal lesions discovered in average-risk women with no acute symptoms. When multiple or bilateral lesions are encountered, each lesion should be characterized separately, and the management is driven by the lesion with the highest score. For risk stratification, the ORADS-MRI system uses five categories (ORADS 1–5), from normal (1) to high risk of malignancy (5) **(Figs. 3 and 4)**.[24]

TREATMENT

The mainstay of treatment in women with a diagnosis of ovarian malignancy is surgical. In oncology centers with special training in minimally invasive surgery, laparoscopy within bag removal of the mass may be done but spillage however small can lead to upstaging of the disease and affect survival.[25] Every effort should be made to achieve maximum cytoreduction of the disease in pelvis as well as upper abdomen and retroperitoneum.

In stage I-IV disease, if optimal cytoreduction is achievable, total hysterectomy and salpingo-oophorectomy along with comprehensive surgical staging and debulking should be performed primarily. This can

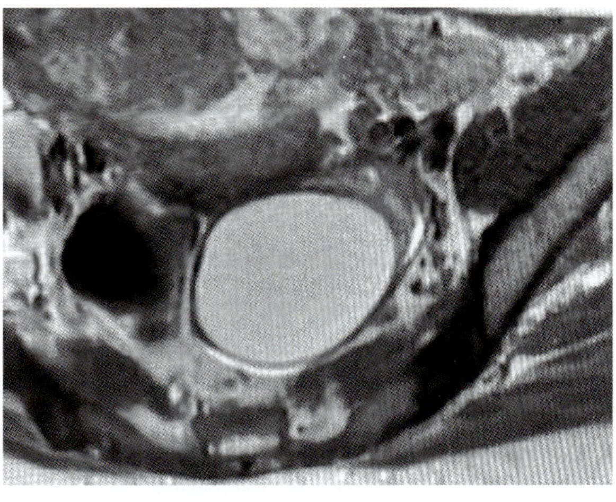

Fig. 3: *ORADS-MRI 2:* Unilocular cyst with no enhancing solid tissue (almost certainly benign).

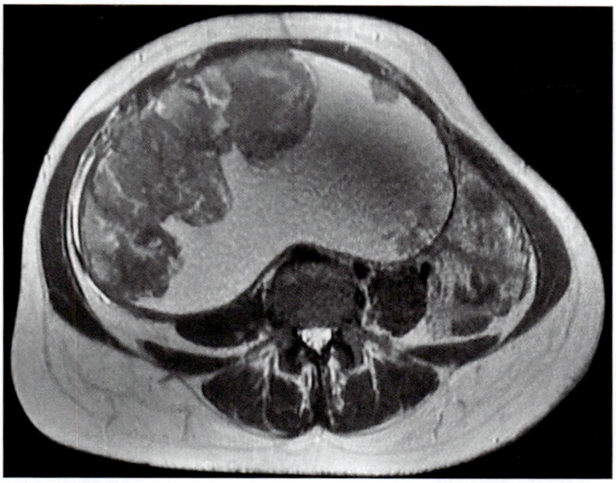

Fig. 4: *ORADS-MRI 5:* Lesion with solid tissue with ascites.

include peritonectomy, bowel resections, visceral resections and total omentectomy. This should be followed by adjuvant chemotherapy after the pathological staging and grading of the disease. If optimal debulking cannot be achieved, the patients should be considered for platinum-based neoadjuvant chemotherapy followed by interval debulking surgery.

In stage II-IV disease, if the response to this primary treatment has been complete, maintenance therapy with PARP inhibitors such as Olaparib, Niraparib or Rucaparib can be given. VEGF inhibitors such as bevacizumab when started during primary platinum-based chemotherapy, can be continued during the maintenance phase along with PARP inhibitors.[3] Various trials have studied the use of targeted agents in BRCA mutation or homologous recombination deficiency. The use of these targeted therapies has significantly improved the progression free survival than chemotherapy alone.[26]

In stage IA if patients are desirous to retain fertility, unilateral salpingo-oophorectomy along with comprehensive surgical staging can be done. In stage IB, bilateral salpingo-oophorectomy with uterine preservation for future assisted reproductive techniques may be considered.[3] Serum AMH and antral follicle count of normal ovary must be done and documented as chemotherapeutic agents can cause a decline in ovarian reserve.

In malignant germ cell tumors, special consideration to fertility sparing is given due to early stage of disease, young age of onset and excellent chemosensitivity of these tumors. Fertility counseling is essential in these young women. Unilateral salpingo-oophorectomy along with limited surgical staging can be done even in advanced stages and followed by Bleomycin, Etoposide, Cisplatin-based chemotherapy for 3–4 cycles. Pediatric age, ill patients with poor performance status can be given the option of low-dose induction chemotherapy with Etoposide Cisplatin to reduce the toxicity.

CONCLUSION

Every effort must be made to distinguish benign from malignant tumors preoperatively, especially before laparoscopic surgery to avoid spillage of tumor cells and upstaging of disease. MRI imaging using ORADS classification is a useful tool to determine when to refer a patient to specialized oncology centers. Survival rates of epithelial ovarian tumors have improved markedly because of radicality of surgery with effective adjuvant chemo- and immunotherapy. Fertility-sparing surgery and fertility counseling must be offered to all young women with germ cell/sex cord stromal tumors. Ovarian reserve must be documented before and after surgery.

REFERENCES

1. Somasegar S, Reddy RA, Karam A. 32 Trends in ovarian cancer incidence and incidence-based mortality: a 15-year population-based analysis. Gynecol Oncol Rep. 2023;48(1):S18.
2. Lim CK, Kim DY, Cho A, Choi JY, Park JY, Kim YM. Role of minimally invasive surgery in early ovarian cancer. Gland Surg. 2021;10(3):1252-9.
3. NCCN 2024; Ovarian Cancer including Fallopian Tube Cancer and Primary Peritoneal Carcinoma. *www.nccn.org. https://www.nccn.org/guidelines/category_1. Accessed on September 28th, 2024.*
4. Giannini A, Di Dio C, Di Donato V, D'oria O, Salerno MG, G Capablo et al. PARP Inhibitors in newly diagnosed and recurrent ovarian cancer. Am J Clin Oncol. 2023;46(9):414-9.
5. Bray F, Laversanne M, Sung H, Ferlay J, Siegel RL, Soerjomataram I, et al. Global cancer statistics 2022: GLOBOCAN estimates of incidence and mortality worldwide for 36 cancers in 185 countries. CA Cancer J Clin. 2024;74(3):229-63.
6. SEER Cancer Statistics Factsheets. Ovary cancer. (2024) Bethesda, MD National Cancer Institute. Available at *https://seer.cancer.gov/statfacts/html/ovary.html.* Accessed on September 24th, 2024.
7. Adhikari L, Hassell LA. WHO classification. PathologyOutlines.com website. *https://www.pathologyoutlines.com/topic/ovarytumorwhoclassif.html.* Accessed on September 23rd, 2024.
8. Goulvent T, Ray-Coquard I, Borel S, Haddad V, Devouassoux-Shisheboran M, Vacher-Lavenu M-C, et al. DICER1 and FOXL2 mutations in ovarian sex cord–stromal tumours: a GINECO Group study. Histopathology. 2016;68(2):279-85.
9. Berek JS, Renz M, Kehoe S, Kumar L, Friedlander M. Cancer of the ovary, fallopian tube, and peritoneum: 2021 update. Int J Gynecol Obstet. 2021;155(1):61-85.
10. Berek JS, Hacker NF, Barile G, Berek D . Berek & Hacker's Gynecologic Oncology, 7th edition. Philadelphia, Wolters Kluwer 2020. pp.1080-98.
11. Sun Y, Liu G. Endometriosis-associated ovarian clear cell carcinoma: a special entity? J Cancer. 2021;12(22):6773-86.
12. Jonsson Sarah, H Jonsson, E Lundin, Christel H, A Idahl. Pelvic inflammatory disease and risk of epithelial ovarian cancer: a national population-based case-control study in Sweden. Am J Obstet Gynecol. 2024;230(1):75.e1-75.e15.

13. Biglia N, Sgandurra P, Bounous VE, Maggiorotto F, Piva E, Pivetta E, et al. Ovarian cancer in *BRCA1* and *BRCA2* gene mutation carriers: analysis of prognostic factors and survival. Ecancermedicalscience. 2016;10:639.
14. Lim AWW, Mesher D, Gentry-Maharaj A, Balogun N, Jacobs I, Menon U. Predictive value of symptoms for ovarian cancer: comparison of symptoms reported by questionnaire, interview, and general practitioner notes. J Natl Cancer Inst. 2012;104(2):114-24.
15. Charkhchi P, Cybulski C, Gronwald J, Wong FO, Narod SA, Akbari MR. CA125 and ovarian cancer: a comprehensive review. Cancers (Basel). 2020;12(12):3730.
16. Matsas A, Stefanoudakis D, Troupis T, Kontzoglou K, Eleftheriades M, Christopoulos P, et al. Tumour markers and their diagnostic significance in ovarian cancer. Life (Basel). 2023;13(8):1689.
17. Lertkhachonsuk AA, Buranawongtrakoon S, Lekskul N, Rermluk N, Wee-Stekly WW, Charakorn C. Serum CA19-9, CA-125 and CEA as tumor markers for mucinous ovarian tumors. J Obstet Gynaecol Res. 2020;46:2287-91.
18. Panici PB, Muzii L, Palaia I, Natalina Manci, Filippo Bellati, Francesco Plotti, et al. Minilaparotomy versus laparoscopy in the treatment of benign adnexal cysts: a randomized clinical study. Eur J Obstet Gynecol Reprod Biol. 2007;133(2):218-22.
19. Royal College of Obstetrician and Gynecologist Greentop Guideline No 34. Jul 2016.
20. Aktürk E, Karaca RE, Alanbay I, Dede M, Karaşahin E, MC Yenen, et al. Comparison of four malignancy risk indices in the detection of malignant ovarian masses. J Gynecol Oncol. 2011;22(3):177-82.
21. Lee SJ, Oh HR, Na S, Hwang HS, Lee SM. Ultrasonographic ovarian mass scoring system for predicting malignancy in pregnant women with ovarian mass. Obstet Gynecol Sci. 2022;65(1):1-13.
22. Andreotti RF, Timmerman D, Strachowski LM, Froyman W, Benacerraf BR, Bennett GL, et al. O-RADS US Risk Stratification and Management System: A Consensus Guideline from the ACR Ovarian-Adnexal Reporting and Data System Committee. Radiology. 2020;294(1):168-85.
23. Timmerman D, Planchamp F, Bourne T, Landolfo C, du Bois A, Chiva L, et al. ESGO/ISUOG/IOTA/ESGE Consensus Statement on preoperative diagnosis of ovarian tumors. Int J Gynecol Cancer. 2021;31:961–82.
24. Pereira PN, Yoshida A, Sarian LO, Barros RHO, Jales RM, Sophie D. Assessment of the performance of the O-RADS MRI score for the evaluation of adnexal masses, with technical notes. Radiol Bras. 2022;55(3):137-44.
25. Falcetta FS, Lawrie TA, Medeiros LR, da Rosa MI, Edelweiss MI, Stein AT, et al. Laparoscopy versus laparotomy for FIGO stage I ovarian cancer. Cochrane Database Syst Rev. 2016;10(10):CD005344.
26. Chiang YC, Lin PH, Cheng WF. Homologous recombination deficiency assays in epithelial ovarian cancer: current status and future direction. Front Oncol. 2021;11:675972.

5 CHAPTER

Persistent Unruptured Ovarian Cyst: How to Proceed?

Rashmi Bagga, Anil E

INTRODUCTION

In the modern day, women as part of cancer screening and contraceptive counseling are subjected to pelvic imaging and physical examination, leading to diagnoses of several cases of ovarian cysts or adnexal masses. The majority are benign and may not require surgery. They are most commonly seen in reproductive years. The actual prevalence is unknown. The chance of women undergoing surgery for suspected ovarian neoplasm in the USA is 5–10% in their whole lifespan. The incidence of ovarian cancer is 10 per 100,000 with a mortality of 6 per 100,000.[1] The characterization of the cyst is important for appropriate treatment. The risk factors for ovarian cyst include age, infertility treatment, use of tamoxifen, pregnancy, hypothyroidism, cigarette smoking, tubal ligation (Functional cysts).[2]

EVALUATION

The main aim of the evaluation is to assess for any signs of malignancy. A detailed medical history along with symptoms and risk factors for ovarian malignancy has to be taken. Any family history of breast/ovarian/bowel cancer has to be noted. Genetic counseling has to be advised in women with a significant family history. A detailed physical examination along with a pelvic exam is needed. A pelvis ultrasound (USG) is the most preferred initial imaging of choice in the evaluation of an ovarian cyst. Transvaginal ultrasound (TVS) with color flow mapping is usually preferred over the transabdominal route. Transabdominal USG is generally done in larger masses extending beyond the pelvis. If advanced imaging is necessary when in doubt about the origin of the cyst, then an MRI can be undertaken **(Table 1)**.

Role of Serum Biomarkers

Serum biomarkers are easily available, cost-effective, and noninvasive tests for identification of malignancy in ovarian cysts. Till date, no serum marker can accurately distinguish benign from malignant lesions. These can only

TABLE 1: USG/Pelvic findings in benign and malignant ovarian tumors.

Clinical features	*Benign*	*Malignant*
Unilateral	+++	+
Bilateral	+	+++
Cystic	+++	–
Solid/fixed	–/–	++/+++
Mobile	+++	–
Irregular	+	+++
Smooth	+++	–
Ascites/cul-de-sac nodules/ rapid growth	–	+++/+++/+++

predict the potential risk of malignancy and are helpful in follow-up and recurrence.

CA-125: It is the most commonly used biomarker in ovarian malignancy. It is usually elevated in 80% of non-mucinous epithelial ovarian cancers but in only 50% of stage I cancer. It has limited specificity and sensitivity as it is also elevated in conditions with peritoneal/serosal inflammation or infection (e.g., tuberculosis and endometriosis) usually seen in premenopausal women. So, CA-125 is unreliable to characterize the cyst in premenopausal women. It is more sensitive to differentiating ovarian cysts as benign or malignant in postmenopausal women and is also included in the RMI score.

HE4: It is expressed in the female genital tract and respiratory tract but not in the ovarian epithelium. HE4 is mainly expressed in serous and endometroid ovarian cancers. Some studies show increased HE4 in 92% of ovarian cancers. It helps to identify patients who are at high risk for platinum resistance. HE4 combined with CA-125 has better prognostic potential in ovarian malignancies. It was shown that a combination of CA-125, HE4, and CT-scan has more predictability of residual disease after neoadjuvant chemotherapy (NACT).[3]

CA 19-9: It is elevated in the gastrointestinal, pancreas, biliary tract, or ovarian tumors, predominantly in mucinous tumors. Though the values are raised in benign gynecological conditions, Cho and Kyung showed that it was much more elevated in borderline and malignant mucinous tumors.[4] In many primary ovarian neoplasms, CA 19-9 is elevated more than CA-125. Abnormally high values are usually seen in malignant tumors.

CEA (carcinoembryonic antigen): It is the most widely used tumor marker for the management of colorectal cancer. It is elevated in 50% of ovarian adenocarcinomas and more than 80% in mucinous types.[5] It may be useful in specific cases to differentiate between primary ovarian cancer and secondary ovarian tumors. There is not enough evidence to include this in the routine initial assessment of ovarian masses.

Other markers: In women less than 40 years age with adnexal masses, measurement of alpha-fetoprotein (AFP), lactate dehydrogenase (LDH), Inhibin B and human chorionic gonadotropin (hCG) helps as there is more prevalence of germ cell tumors in this age group.

HOW TO DIFFERENTIATE FROM A MALIGNANT OVARIAN MASS?

Risk of malignancy index (RMI): The RMI provides a method to differentiate benign masses from malignant ones. It includes menopausal status, CA-125, and transvaginal ultrasound (TVS) scores. Though many variants of RMI have been developed, RMI-1 is most studied and a score cut-off ≥200 has a sensitivity and specificity of 78 and 87% respectively.[6]

International Ovarian Tumor Analysis Group (IOTA) rules: This group used simple USG features to differentiate benign (B-rules) from malignant masses (M-rules) with a sensitivity and specificity of 92% and 96% respectively.[7] They are classified as benign if any of B features are present. If a woman has any of M features, she is further evaluated for malignancy. If no features are observed, then it is deemed inconclusive.

Pattern recognition: Certain abnormalities are obvious with simple descriptors. These are shown in **Box 1 and Table 2**.

Ovarian-Adnexal Reporting and Data System (O-RADS): This USG-based scoring system increases sensitivity and negative predictive value, opting for more conservative management for benign features and evaluation and oncology referral in patients with malignant features **(Table 3)**.

ORADS-MRI score increases specificity and positive predictive value for detecting malignancy[8] **(Table 4)**.

BOX 1: *Pattern recognition:* Certain abnormalities are obvious with simple descriptors.

- *Endometrioma:* Unilocular tumor with ground-glass echogenicity in premenopausal women
- *Simple cyst/cystadenoma:* Unilocular tumor with regular walls and less than 10 cm in maximum diameter
- *Functional cyst/ hemorrhagic cyst:* Unilocular tumor with regular walls and no other benign descriptors
- *Benign cystic teratoma or dermoid:* Unilocular tumor with mixed echogenicity and acoustic shadows in premenopausal women
- *Malignant tumor with ascites:* Tumor with ascites and moderate color Doppler blood flow in postmenopausal women

TABLE 2: Difference between B-rules and M-rules.

B-rules	*M-rules*
Unilocular cysts	Irregular solid tumor
The presence of solid components where the largest solid component	Ascites
Presence of acoustic shadowing	At least four papillary structures
Smooth multilocular tumor with the largest diameter	Irregular multilocular solid tumor with largest diameter ≥100 mm
No blood flow	Very strong blood flow

TABLE 3: Ovarian-Adnexal Reporting and Data System (ORADS).

ORADS group	*Ultrasound descriptors*	*Risk of malignancy*
ORADS 0	Incomplete evaluation	Not stated
ORADS 1	Normal premenopausal ovary	0%
ORADS 2	• Classic hemorrhagic cyst ≥5 to <10 cm • Classic dermoid cyst <10 cm • Classic endometrioma <10 cm • Unilocular smooth cyst <10 cm • Other unilocular smooth cyst ≥3 to <10 cm	1%
ORADS 3	• Unilocular smooth cyst ≥10 cm • Unilocular irregular wall • Multilocular smooth CS 1–3 <10 cm • Solid smooth CS 1	1 to <10%
ORADS 4	• Multilocular smooth >10 cm CS 1–3 • Multilocular smooth CS 4 • Multilocular irregular • Unilocular-solid no papillary projections • Unilocular-solid 1–3 papillary projections • Multilocular-solid CS 1–2 • Solid smooth CS 2–3	10 to <50%
ORADS 5	• Unilocular-solid with >4 papillary projections • Multilocular-solid CS 3–4 • Solid smooth CS 4 • Solid irregular • Ascites or metastases	50–100%

What is the Role of MRI in Adnexal Lesions?

MRI is advised when we need a more specific diagnosis and in conditions, where:

1. The origin of the lesion has to be confirmed.
2. The lesion is more than 10 cm.
3. If the tumor contains solid components and further characterization of mass is required.

TABLE 4: ORADS-MRI score.

ORADS-MRI score	*Risk category*	*Positive predictive value for malignancy*	*Lexicon description*
0	Incomplete evaluation	N/A	N/A
1	Normal ovaries	N/A	• No ovarian lesion • A follicle is defined as a simple cyst ≤3 cm • A hemorrhagic cyst is ≤3 cm • Corpus luteum ≤3 cm. All of the above is in pre-menopausal women
2	Almost certainly benign	<0.5%	• Unilocular cyst (any fluid content) with no enhancing wall and solid tissue or • Unilocular cyst (simple or endometriotic fluid) with enhancing wall and no enhancing solid tissue • A lesion with lipid content or para-ovarian cyst with any fluid content and both should not have enhanced solid tissue • Lesion with dark T2/dark DWI solid tissue • Dilated fallopian tube with no enhancing solid tissue
3	Low risk	~5%	• Unilocular cyst (proteinaceous, hemorrhagic, or mucinous fluid) with smooth enhancing wall and no enhancing solid tissue • A multilocular cyst (any fluid content) with smooth septae and wall with enhancement with enhanced solid tissue • Lesion with solid tissue (excluding T2 dark/DWI dark) • Dilated fallopian tube with any type of fluid and no solid tissue enhancement
4	Inter-mediate risk	~50%	• A lesion with solid tissue (excluding T2 dark/DWI dark) • Intermediate risk time intensity curve in DCE MRI • If DCE MRI is not feasible, score 4 is any lesion with solid tissue that is enhancing ≤ myometrium at 30–40s on non-DCE MRI • A lesion with lipid content, large volume enhancing solid tissue

Contd…

Contd...

ORADS-MRI score	*Risk category*	*Positive predictive value for malignancy*	*Lexicon description*
5	High risk	~90%	• A lesion with solid tissue (excluding T2 dark/DWI dark) • High-risk time-intensity curve in DCE-MRI • If DCE-MRI is not feasible, score 5 is any lesion with solid tissue that is enhancing >myometrium at 30–40s on non-DCE MRI • Peritoneal, mesenteric, or omental nodularity or irregular thickening with or without ascites

4. Less experienced gynecological sonologists.

In a study conducted by Rizzo et al., the O-RADS MRI risk score had a sensitivity of 92% and specificity of 91%.[9]

Role of CT Scan in the Evaluation of Adnexal Masses

If an ovarian malignancy is suspected, then it is helpful to look for metastasis, ascites, and lymph node enlargement. It is usually not a part of diagnoses of ovarian masses.

When Should the Women be Referred to an Oncologist?

- Women with a history of infertility, endometriosis and cancer, family history of cancer.
- Patients with adnexal mass have solid areas with strong/central color flow, more than 4 papillary projections (>3 mm), thick multiple irregular septations, ascites, and peritoneal thickening.
- Adnexal masses with indeterminate features in ultrasound can be referred.
- Bilateral masses with clinical and sonological features suggestive of malignancy.[10]
- When CA-125 is greater than 200 in a premenopausal woman or if RMI is >200.

MANAGEMENT (OBSERVATION VS SURGERY)

The first thing is to make an appropriate diagnosis based on history, examination, and diagnostic tests. The patient's symptomology also has to be considered to decide if surgery is necessary. Opinions from other specialists are sometimes needed for further management. If the decision for surgery has been taken after assessing the cyst, then you have to decide the route of surgery (Open vs. minimally invasive). Patients kept under observation need timely spaced repeat USG.

Management in pre-menopausal women: Functional cysts usually are less than 7 cm, and cysts of size less than 5 cm are benign (95%), these women will be under observation and a repeat scan is done after 6–8 weeks to look for size and cyst characteristics. Ovarian cysts of more than 10 cm are usually treated surgically as the chances of spontaneous resolution are low. Women having ovarian cysts with septa and without solid components are usually non-malignant and can be kept under follow-up.

Management of Adnexal Mass in a Premenopausal Woman[11] (Flowchart 1)

According to some bodies, there is no cut-off for the size of ovarian cysts for surgery.[6] Persistent ovarian cysts and cysts which increase in size are seldom functional. Minimally invasive surgery (MIS) (Laparoscopy/Robotic) is advised if the cyst is presumed to be benign irrespective of the size. If the cyst is very large with solid components, then staging laparotomy is required. The route of surgery is dependent on factors like, the fitness of the woman for laparoscopy, characteristics of the cysts, and surgeon skills. Aspiration of the cyst has a high rate of recurrence and is not recommended. Spillage should be avoided during surgery as cysts cannot be considered benign before surgery. If the cyst is ruptured, then thorough peritoneal lavage has to be done. Ovarian preservation has been in practice for benign lesions. Unilateral oophorectomy has no effects on menstruation and pregnancy rates.

Management in postmenopausal women: Patients with normal CA-125 levels and asymptomatic unilocular cysts of less than 5 cm in size can be left for observation with frequent USG follow-up and CA-125 testing

Flowchart 1: Management of adnexal mass in a premenopausal woman.

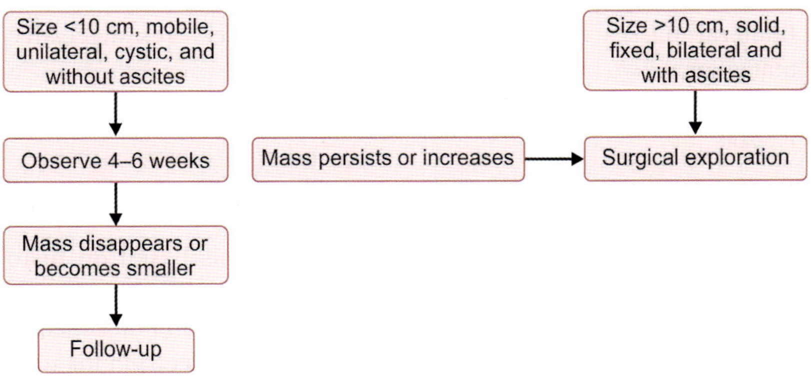

BOX 2: *Adnexal masses:* Indications for surgery.[11]

- Persistent ovarian cyst for 6–8 weeks and of >5 cm in size
- Solid ovarian lesion
- Ovarian cyst with papillary vegetation on the cyst wall
- Adnexal mass greater than 10 cm in size
- Ascites
- Palpable adnexal mass in premenarchal or postmenopausal patient
- Torsion or if there is a cyst rupture

every 3-6 months.[6,11] Any suspicion of malignancy, complex cysts, and cysts with RMI >200 should undergo surgery. If the surgeon has planned for MIS, extra care has to be taken in suspicion of malignancy and raised CA-125 levels with a facility for intraoperative frozen section. The consent has to be taken for conversion to laparotomy and performed by an experienced surgeon **(Box 2)**.

SUMMARY

- Most of the ovarian cysts are benign, but malignancy has to be ruled out.
- Biochemical markers alone cannot differentiate between benign and malignant cysts.
- Imaging features plus biomarkers help in the diagnosis of malignant masses.

REFERENCES

1. NIH NCI Cancer Stat Facts Ovarian Cancer. https://seer.cancer.gov/statfacts/html/ovary.html. Published 2022. Accessed September 29, 2022.
2. Mobeen S, Apostol R. Ovarian Cyst. [Updated 2023 Jun 5]. In: StatPearls [Internet]. Treasure Island (FL): StatPearls Publishing; 2024 Jan-.
3. Anastasi E, Farina A, Granato T, Colaiacovo F, Pucci B, Tartaglione S, et al. Recent insight about HE4 Role in ovarian cancer oncogenesis. Int J Mol Sci. 2023;24(13):10479. doi: 10.3390/ijms241310479. PMID: 37445657; PMCID: PMC10341457.
4. Pyeon SY, Park JY, Ki KD, Lee JM. Abnormally high level of CA-19-9 in a benign ovarian cyst. Obstet Gynecol Sci. 2015;58(6):530-2. doi: 10.5468/ogs.2015.58.6.530. Epub 2015 Nov 16. PMID: 26623421; PMCID: PMC4663235.
5. Sagi-Dain L, Lavie O, Auslander R, Sagi S. CEA in evaluation of adnexal mass: retrospective cohort analysis and review of the literature. Int J Biol Markers. 2015;30(4):e394-400. doi: 10.5301/jbm.5000158. PMID: 26109367.
6. Practice Bulletin No. 174: Evaluation and management of adnexal masses. Obstet Gynecol. 2016;128(5):e210-e226. doi: 10.1097/AOG.00000000000000
7. Tantipalakorn C, Wanapirak C, Khunamornpong S, Sukpan K, Tongsong T. IOTA simple rules in differentiating between benign and malignant ovarian tumours. Asian Pac J Cancer Prev. 2014;15(13):5123-16.
8. Sadowski EA, Rockall A, Thomassin-Naggara I, Barroilhet LM, Wallace SK, Jha P, et al. Adnexal Lesion Imaging: Past, Present, and Future. Radiology.

2023;307(5):e223281. doi: 10.1148/radiol.223281. Epub 2023 May 9. PMID: 37158725.

9. Rizzo S, Cozzi A, Dolciami M, et al. ORADS-MRI: a systematic review and meta-analysis of diagnostic performance and category-wise malignancy rates. Radiology. 2022. 10.1148/radiol.220795. Published online November 22, 2022.
10. Salvador S, Scott S, Glanc P, Eiriksson L, Jang J-H, Sebastianelli A, et al. 403: Initial investigation and management of adnexal masses. J Obstet Gynaecol Can. 2020;42(8):1021.e3–1029.e3.
11. Washington C, Gunderson CC, Mannel RS. Adnexal masses. In: Creasman WT, Mannel RS, Mutch DG, Tewari K (Eds). Disaia and Creasman Textbook of Clinical Gynecologic Oncology, 10th edn. Philadelphia: Elsevier; 2023. pp. 229-50.

SECTION 3

Endometrial Cancer: Red Flag

6. **New FIGO Classification of Endometrial Cancer**
   Seema Singhal, Meenal Bhati, Sholanki Haldar
7. **Screening for Endometrial Cancer**
   Geetha Balsarkar
8. **Lynch Syndrome**
   Mala Srivastava, Saloni Chadha
9. **Radical Hysterectomy: The Wertheim's Surgery**
   Samar Gupte

6

CHAPTER

New FIGO Classification of Endometrial Cancer

Seema Singhal, Meenal Bhati, Sholanki Haldar

INTRODUCTION

Historically, staging systems of endometrial carcinoma by FIGO staging systems have been "clinical." The first "surgico-pathological" staging system was introduced in 1988, which was followed for two decades. Although the year of 2009 embarked updated staging of cervical, vulvar and novel staging for uterine sarcomas, yet FIGO 2009 staging was purely established on anatomy and revision changes were relatively limited. Peritoneal washings were removed from the staging system and cervical stromal involvement was separately recognized.[1]

Since the 2009 FIGO staging, many advancements have progressed in the spectrum of pathology, including molecular subtypes of endometrial carcinoma. The Cancer Genome Atlas project (2013) applied in-depth genomic, proteomic, and transcriptomic methodologies to a cohort of 373 endometrioid and serous endometrial carcinomas and exhibited clarity on the diverse biological nature of endometrial cancers and contrastive prognostic outcomes. Hence, the "modern" molecular classification marked the era of paradigm shift to precision medicine and has been adapted and integrated into the new FIGO 2023 Staging System.[2]

The system aims to achieve better definition of the respective prognostic groups and create substations that indicate more appropriate treatment strategies, encompassing surgical, radiation, and systemic therapies.

ALTERATIONS FROM TRADITIONAL STAGING SYSTEM

Through the course of time, AJCC staging has gradually shifted to staging systems which include histologic prognostic factors, biomarkers, and molecular details, e.g., in breast, head and neck, prostatic carcinomas. It needs to be appreciated that gynecologic malignancies are the only cancers not staged by TNM staging, although. Therefore, the need of the hour lies in a system analogous to other malignancies, such as, breast cancer, where all staging categories are blended with non-anatomic or molecular data, to create the final stage. Hence, this transition should provide a comprehensive analysis, leading to improved prognostication and clinical decisions **(Table 1)**.

TABLE 1: Molecular and clinicopathological features of endometrial cancer molecular subgroups.[3,4]

	POLEmut (i.e., POLE exonculease domain mutation)	*dMMR (i.e., MSI)*	*NSMP (i.e., p53-wt)*	*p53 aberrant*
Prevalence in TCGA cohort	5–15%	25–30%	30–40%	5–15%
Associated molecular features	>100 mut/Mb, SCNA—very low, MSS	10–100 mut/Mb, SCNA—low, MSI	<10 mut/Mb, SCNA—low, MSS	<10 mut/Mb, SCNA—high, MSS
Most frequent-histological features	• Endometrioid • Often high grade • Ambiguous morphology • Prominent TILs and TLSs	• Endometrioid • Often high-grade • LVSI substantial • Prominent TILs • MELF-type invasion	• Mostly low grade • Notable absence of TILs • Squamous differentiation • ER/PgR diffuse	• All histological subtypes • Mostly high grade • High cytonuclear atypia • Low level TILs
Associated clinical features	• Lower BMI • Early stage (IA–IB) • Early onset	• Higher BMI • Lynch syndrome	Higher BMI	• Lower BMI • Advanced stage • Late onset
Diagnostic test	*NGS/Sanger/Hotspot:* P286R, V411L, S297F, A456P, S459F	*MMR-IHC:* MLH1, MSH2, MSH6, PMS2; MSI assay		p53 IHC Mutant-like/abnormal staining
Prognosis	Excellent	Intermediate	• Intermediate • Stage-dependent	Poor

TOP TIER FIGO 2023 STAGING CHANGES[5]

- Integrated approach with histological subtypes, inclusive of tumor type, tumor grade and nuances of lymphovascular space invasion (LVSI) to result in the accuracy of staging
- Incorporation of molecular profile into staging of carcinoma
- Modification of stage according to anatomical spread (adnexa, cervix, pelvic and abdominal peritoneum)
- Distinguished, separate entities between synchronous and metastatic endometrial and ovarian primary
- Detailed description of nodal involvement; significant impact on classification of sentinel lymph node classification (micrometastasis vs macrometastasis)
- Elaborate and scrupulous distinction of stage III and IV disease to better represent the clinical scenario, derive prognostication and enable a more appropriate and refined decision-making **(Table 2)**.

TABLE 2: FIGO 2023 Staging of Carcinoma Endometrium.[5]

Stage	*Description*
Stage I	Confined to the uterine corpus and ovary
IA	Disease limited to the endometrium OR non-aggressive histological type, i.e., low-grade endometroid, with <50% MI, with no or focal lymphovascular space involvement (LVSI) OR good prognosis disease
IA1	Non-aggressive histological type limited to an endometrial polyp OR confined to the endometrium
IA2	Non-aggressive histological types involving less than half of the myometrium with no or focal LVSI
IA3	Low-grade endometrioid carcinomas limited to the uterus and ovary
IB	Non-aggressive histological types with invasion of half or more of the myometrium, and with no or focal LVSI
IC	Aggressive histological types limited to a polyp or confined to the endometrium
Stage II	Invasion of cervical stroma with extrauterine extension OR with substantial LVSI OR aggressive histological types with myometrial invasion
IIA	Invasion of the cervical stroma of non-aggressive histological types
IIB	Substantial LVSI of non-aggressive histological types
IIC	Aggressive histological types with any myometrial involvement
Stage III	Local and/or regional spread of the tumor of any histological subtype
IIIA	Invasion of uterine serosa, adnexa, or both by direct extension or metastasis: • *IIIA1:* Spread to ovary or fallopian tube (except when meeting stage IA3 criteria) • *IIIA2:* Involvement of uterine subserosa or spread through the uterine serosa

Contd...

Contd...

Stage	*Description*
IIIB	Metastasis or direct spread to the vagina and/or to the parametria or pelvic peritoneum: • *IIIB1:* Metastasis or direct spread to the vagina and/or the parametria • *IIIB2:* Metastasis to the pelvic peritoneum
IIIC	Metastasis to the pelvic or para-aortic lymph nodes or both: • *IIIC1:* Metastasis to the pelvic lymph nodes • *IIIC1(i):* Micrometastasis • *IIIC1(ii):* Macrometastasis • *IIIC2:* Metastasis to para-aortic lymph nodes up to the renal vessels, with or without metastasis to the pelvic lymph nodes • *IIIC2i:* Micrometastasis • *IIIC2ii:* Macrometastasis
Stage IV	Spread to the bladder mucosa and/or intestinal mucosa and/or distance metastasis
IVA	Invasion of the bladder mucosa and/or the intestinal/bowel mucosa
IVB	Abdominal peritoneal metastasis beyond the pelvis
IVC	Distant metastasis, including metastasis to any extra- or intra-abdominal lymph nodes above the renal vessels, lungs, liver, brain, or bone

HISTOLOGY

Tumor Type

The revised FIGO 2023 staging includes the recent 5th WHO classification, published in 2020 and includes designated subtypes that would have implications in predicting respective prognosis. Histological types are broadly divided into aggressive and non-aggressive. Non-aggressive histological types include grade 1 and 2 endometrial endometrioid carcinomas (EEC), also the most common type encountered. Aggressive histologies include high-grade (grade 3) EEC, serous carcinoma (SC), clear cell carcinoma (CCC), mixed carcinoma (MC), undifferentiated carcinoma (UC), carcinosarcoma (CS), gastrointestinal type and mesonephric-like mucinous carcinomas.[5,6]

The high-grade EEC (grade 3) has benefited the most from applying molecular classification, which is into four subgroups:[7-10]

1. p53 abnormal, based on mutant-like immunostaining (p53abn)
2. MMR deficient, based on loss of mismatch repair protein expression (MMRd)
3. Presence of POLE exonuclease domain hotspot mutation (POLE)
4. No specific molecular profile (NSMP), in which none of these molecular aberrations were present

POLEmut in early-stage disease comes under good prognosis, p53 abnormal (p53abn) from a bad prognosis group, no-specific molecular profile

(NSMP) group with estrogen receptor (ER)-negative has bad prognosis. Also to note, in mismatch repair deficient (MMRd) molecular subtype, grading does not hold any relevance.[5,11-13]

Tumor Grade

The role of histological grade is very important in EEC and in NSMP, whereas the other histology types like SC, CCC, MC, UC, CS, and mesonephric-like and gastrointestinal mucinous type carcinomas are considered high-grade by definition. The binary approach of grading by WHO Classification of Tumors, Female Genital Tumors has been included in the revised FIGO staging scheme. In low-grade EECs, grade 1 and 2 tumors are included, which exhibit up to 5% and 6–50% solid non-glandular growth respectively, whereas in high-grade EECs (grade 3) exhibit 50% or more solid component. The role of three-tiered system role holds paramount importance for patients requesting and eligible for fertility-preserving strategies. In grade 1 or 2 tumor if nuclear atypia is excessive for the grade, it raises the grade by one.[5,6,13]

Cervical stromal invasion: It is defined as any invasion of the cervical stroma, at the level of or beyond than a benign endocervical crypt. Due to high interobserver variation in reporting this strict criteria should be followed.[1,5,14]

Adnexal involvement: Adnexal involvement is important in overall survival of endometrial cancers. The revised 2023 FIGO staging for endometrial carcinoma includes Stage IA3 when the following criteria are met in a low-grade EEC: (1) No more than superficial myometrial invasion is present (<50%); (2) The absence of substantial LVSI; (3) The absence of additional metastases; (4) The ovarian tumor is unilateral, limited to the ovary, without capsule invasion/breach (equivalent to pT1a). The cases not fulfilling these criteria should be interpreted as extensive spread of the endometrial carcinoma to the ovary (Stage IIIA1). Fallopian tube involvement is considered in stage IIIA1.[5,14]

Uterine serosal involvement: ISGyP recommendations are followed while defining uterine serosal involvement that is, tumor reaching up to submesothelial fibroconnective tissue or the mesothelial layer, regardless of whether they are present on the serosal surface of the uterus or not.[5,15-17]

FIGO 2023 mentions that if available and feasible, molecular classification testing is to be encouraged in all endometrial carcinomas. Molecular subtype assignment can be done on a biopsy, and need not be repeated on hysterectomy specimen.

MMRd/NSMP does not modify FIGO stage; holds intermediate prognosis and serve as reference for POLEmut and p53abn tumors.[5,18]

The evolving field in the new staging system is the Multiple Classifiers. For tumors (5%) having combination of more than one molecular feature, classification to be categorized as follows:[5,19,20]

- POLEmut/MMRd + p53abn = retain favorable prognosis of POLEmut/MMRd
- POLEmut + p53abn = POLEmut
- MMRd + p53abn = MMRd
- Pathogenic POLEmut + MMRd = Screening for lynch syndrome
- Stage I/II low-grade endometrioid carcinoma p53abn = Tumor upstaged to IIC2m-p53abn

PIVOTAL CHANGES

Stage shift: Up- or downstaging of stage I and II depending on the molecular profile, *POLE*mut- and p53abn-status.

Implications

In view of the changes in FIGO 2023 staging, the number of patients classified as Stage II would increase.

In an international pooled analysis, Schwameis R, et al. Confirmed substantial substage shifts, but a more accurate prediction of PFS and OS by the 2023 FIGO staging system compared to 2009. Stage shifts occurred in 143/519 (27.6%) patients, with 123 upshifts (23.7%) and 20 (3.9%) downshifts. 2023 FIGO staging system identified a stage I cohort with a notably higher 5-year PFS rate compared to 2009 (93.0% vs. 87.4%, respectively). For stage II disease, the 5-year PFS rate was similar in 2023 and the 2009 FIGO staging systems (70.2% vs. 71.2%, respectively).[21]

The two new molecular defined substages IAm*POLE*mut and IICmp53abn exhibited distinct, particularly favorable and adverse oncologic outcomes within early-stage disease, respectively. A remarkably lower 5-year PFS rate for stage III patients was revealed in the 2023 FIGO staging system compared to 2009 (44.4% vs. 54.1%, respectively).[21]

Myometrial Invasion

The myometrium invasion is noted by overall myometrial thickness infiltrated in percentage by carcinoma using three categories: none; <50%; or ≥50%. The depth of myometrial invasion holds a very important role in prognostication.[5]

Lymphovascular Space Invasion

Recommendation by WHO 2020 has been adapted by this FIGO system to distinguish “substantial” or “extensive” LVSI from “focal” or “no” LVSI where extensive/substantial LVSI is defined when ≥5 vessels are involved, focal LVSI means <5 vessels.[5,6]

In 2019, SweGCG study evaluated 1587 endometrioid endometrial carcinoma patients with known nodal status and study results concluded LVSI to carry five times risk of lymph node metastasis and that, LVSI most important prognostic factor for overall survival in lymph node.[22]

Gian Franco Zannoni, et al. raised some critical issues in reporting the distinct LVSI categories. The authors highlighted lack of well-defined standardizations of "multifocal" or "diffuse" LVSI, that may lead to inconsistency in reporting; significant variation of reported foci of LVSI due to non-standardized number of microscopic sections examined; poor reproducibility among pathologists, leading to inconsistencies in diagnosing LVSI; interpretation of LVSI may be impacted by necrosis and pre-analytical phase issues, affecting accuracy and hence, they concluded the new proposed changes may be "not too soon, but maybe too much".[23]

As the assessment is subjective, retraction artefacts, artefactual LVSI secondary to autolysis/spreading artefact, MELF pattern myometrial invasion mimicking LVSI, may create inconvenience in quantifying LVSI.[24,25]

Although the patients included in PORTEC trial were not evaluated on lymph nodes, a combined analysis of the PORTEC (PORTEC I, II) trials reported that substantial LVSI was diagnosed in approximately 5% of the cohorts and the respective patients experienced a higher rate of locoregional recurrences.[26,27]

To raise the concern if evidence of substantial LVSI is substitute or independent predictor of lymph node positivity, multiple studies have been conducted. Christian Dagher, et al. retrospectively identified patients with FIGO 2009 stage I endometrioid endometrial cancer treated surgically with total hysterectomy and lymph node assessment.[28] Risk of recurrence was aggravated for patients having both focal and substantial LVSI, the entities were not prognostically distinct and on multivariate analysis, any form of LVSI was associated with increased risk of progression/death.[28]

In another retrospective analysis, Aseem Rai Bhatnagar, et al. reported the prognostic impact of substantial LVSI in previously diagnosed Stage I endometrial carcinoma with negative lymph nodes on histopathology. The authors concluded no significant difference in 5-year survival (recurrence-free, disease-specific, or overall), and in the patterns of initial recurrence between patients with focal and substantial LVSI.[29]

Since presence of substantial LVSI, according to current 2023 FIGO staging, upstages any patient to "at least" IIB, ideally, would predict worse outcome in any patient independently. On the contrary, theoretically, for the same patients, who have had complete or maximum lymph node assessment, substantial LVSI would theoretically upstage the disease and likely increase radiation therapy.

TABLE 3: Fertility preservation.

Stage designation	*Molecular finding in early-stage cancer (Stage I and II)*[5]
Stage IAmPOLEmut	*POLEmut* endometrial carcinoma, confined to the uterine corpus or with cervical extension, regardless of the degree of LVSI or histological type
Stage IICmp53abn	p53abn endometrial carcinoma confined to the uterine corpus with any myometrial invasion with or without cervical invasion, and regardless of the degree of LVSI or histological types

Hence, due to resultant stage-shift owing to the latest system, varied consequences may be noted **(Table 3)**.

Stage IA1

Fertility Preservation

Both NCCN and ESGO/ESHRE/ESGE guidelines recommend that fertility sparing therapy in Grade 1, Stage IA noninvasive disease/without myometrial invasion, without genetic risk factors. ESGO adds that binary grading system for endometrial carcinoma should not be implemented in these women.[30,31]

Ovarian preservation may be considered in women <45-year age, without any genetic risk factors.[31]

Stage IA2

In a retrospective series at MSKCC (2020), among 959 patients with Stage I low-grade endometrioid endometrial carcinoma, very low risk of lymph node metastases was reported. Hence, the surgical plan in this category of patients remains the same, that is, assessment of sentinel lymph node would be sufficient, and no restaging would be necessary if done already.[32]

Stage IA3

No fertility preservation can be done in this group; complete staging inclusive of peritoneal assessment, omentectomy, lymphadenectomy needs to be done. Restaging can be considered if not done previously. Precursors to endometrioid carcinoma in the endometrium (atypical hyperplasia) and in the ovary (endometriosis, adenofibroma) are among the criteria for classification of favorable outcome by ISGyP recommendations but not by WHO or 2023 FIGO staging system.[33]

Stage IC

For aggressive histotypes confined within polyp or endometrium, there remains less likelihood of any change in management protocol. Complete staging with hysterectomy, bilateral salpingo-oophorectomy, lymph node staging and omentectomy would be necessary in this cohort and restaging to be considered to avoid implications in adjuvant setting. For patients having no residual disease following surgical staging, NCCN recommends observation.[30]

A study from China was published in 2023, retrospectively reporting outcomes of fertility preservation treatments using molecular classifications based on NGS panel. They reported that *POLE* mutations had the highest disease progression rate (50.0%, $P = 0.013$) and microsatellite instability-high (MSI-H) group had the highest recurrence rate (50.0%, $P = 0.042$).[34]

Therefore, the implementation of molecular classification in this scenario is promising and can aid in selection of appropriate medical regimes to achieve better outcome.

High-grade endometrioid histology has been noted to fall in any of the four molecular subtypes, carry diverse prognosis and hence, would change management strategy.

On the contrary, no methodology has been recommended by FIGO 2023 for molecular subtyping, and the latter may possibly remain unavailable in low-resource settings.

In another study, Bozena Dobrzycka, et al. evaluated the prognosis of Stage I endometrial carcinoma following re-classification by FIGO 2023 staging system. Among 139 patients, Stage IC, aggressive histological types, p53 abnormal protein expression was associated with lower 5-year overall survival.[35]

Stage IIB

This substage harbors increased the likelihood of radiation treatment, especially external beam radiotherapy, due to upstaging of patients.[5]

Stage IICmp53abn

Aggressive histologies with any myometrial invasion are treated with chemotherapy with or without radiation, even following 2009 staging and ESGO/ESTRO/ESP risk stratification system. For endometrioid p53 mutated subtype, it would require to rule out multiple classifiers, pathogenic *POLE* and MMRd prior to providing aggressive adjuvant treatment.[5,36]

Stage IIIA1 and IIIA2

Differentiation between adnexal (IIIA1) and uterine serosa infiltration (IIIA2) can more effectively represent tumor behavior, especially in high-grade and non-endometrioid carcinomas. This 2023 FIGO system introduces the concept of "uterine subserosa" (IIIA2), not previously defined otherwise.[5]

Stage IIIB2

Separately recognizes disease in pelvic peritoneum, previously designated as IVB. With disseminated disease above Stage III, surgical staging and adjuvant treatment protocol remain unchanged.[5]

Different substaging of Stage III aim to better reflect clinical decisions in respect to surgical versus non-surgical first-line treatments for advanced stage disease. These management startegies are expected to vary significantly in cases with limited pelvic versus extensive/extrapelvic peritoneal carcinomatosis.

Lymph Node Status

TNM classification of malignant tumor cells is followed in this system, defining macrometastases as 2 mm, micrometastases as >0.2–2 mm and/or >200 cells, and isolated tumor cells are up to 0.2 mm in size and up to 200 cells. Ultrastaging is recommended for the analysis of sentinel lymph nodes.[5] This subcategorization allows enhanced identification of small volume disease, including micrometastasis, in ultrastaged sentinel lymph node.

A very recent study was published in 2024, that explored molecular subtyping in patients with endometrioid endometrial cancer and isolated tumor cells or node negative disease. Molecular classification was not found to have a significant association with the presence of isolated tumor cells, although the copy number-high/TP53 abnormal subtype was a poor prognostic indicator, even in early-stage disease.[37]

Another prospective PROME trial (2024) concluded that molecular classification does not seem useful to tailor the need of nodal dissection in apparent early-stage endometrial carcinoma. Although, p53 abnormality predicts risk of having advanced disease at presentation.[38]

Therefore, summarizing the few drawbacks or challenges met with new FIGO 2023 staging system:

- Too many changes and multiple subcategorizations to be implemented in practical management by clinicians and pathologists
- Considerable interobserver variability in respect to few parameters
- Close resemblance to the ESGO/ESTRO/ESP risk-stratification system using molecular classification; "staging" almost made equivalent to 'risk stratification"
- Possible multiple changes of primarily assigned disease stage, during the course of management of any patient.

REFERENCES

1. Abu-Rustum NR, Zhou Q, Iasonos A, et al. The Revised 2009 FIGO Staging System for Endometrial Cancer: Should the 1988 FIGO Stages IA and IB Be Altered? Int J Gynecol Cancer. 2011;21:511-6.

2. Levine D. The Cancer Genome Atlas Research Network. Integrated genomic characterization of endometrial carcinoma. Nature. 2013;497:67-73.
3. Oaknin A, et al. Endometrial cancer: ESMO Clinical Practice Guideline for diagnosis, treatment and follow-up. Ann Oncol. 2022;33(9):860-77.
4. Léon-Castillo A. Update in the molecular classification of endometrial carcinoma. Int J Gynecol Cancer. 2023;33(3):333-42.
5. Berek JS, Matias-Guiu X, Creutzberg C, et al. FIGO staging of endometrial cancer. Int J Gynecol Obstet. 2023;162:383-94. doi:10.1002/ijgo.14923.
6. WHO Classification of Tumours Editorial Board. Female Genital Tumours, WHO Classification of Tumours (Vol 4), 5th edition. IARC Press; 2020.
7. Corr B, Cosgrove C, Spinosa D, et al. Endometrial cancer: molecular classification and future treatments. BMJ Medicine. 2022;1:e000152. doi: 10.1136/bmjmed-2022-000152.
8. Bosse T, Nout RA, McAlpine JN, et al. Molecular classification of grade 3 endometrioid endometrial cancers identifies distinct prognostic subgroups. Am J Surg Pathol. 2018;42(5):561-8.
9. Barlin JN, Soslow RA, Lutz M, et al. Redefining stage I endometrial cancer: incorporating histology, a binary grading system, myometrial invasion, and lymph node assessment. Int J Gynecol Cancer. 2013;23(9):1620-8.
10. Jamieson A, Huvila J, Chiu D, et al. Grade and estrogen receptor expression identify a subset of no specific profile endometrial carcinomas at a very low risk of disease specific death. Mod Pathol. 2023;36(4):100212. doi:10.1016/j.modpat.2022.100085
11. Colombo N, Creutzberg C, Amant F, et al. ESMO-ESGO-ESTRO consensus conference on endometrial cancer: diagnosis, treatment and follow-up. Ann Oncol. 2016;27(1):16-41.
12. Vermij L, Jobson JJ, Leon-Castillo A, et al. Prognostic refinement of NSMP high-risk endometrial cancers using oestrogen receptor immunohistochemistry. Brit J Cancer. 2023;128:1360-8. doi:10.1038/s41416-023-02141-0.
13. Soslow RA, Tornos C, Park KJ, et al. Endometrial carcinoma diagnosis: use of FIGO grading and genomic subcategories in clinical practice: recommendations of the International Society of Gynecological Pathologists. Int J Gynecol Pathol. 2019;38(Suppl 1): S64-S74.
14. Creasman WT, Morrow CP, Bundy BN, Homesley HD, Graham JE, Heller PB. Surgical pathologic spread patterns of endometrial cancer: a gynecologic oncology group study. Cancer. 1987;60(8 Suppl):2035-41.
15. Lindauer J, Fowler JM, Manolitsas TP, et al. Is there a prognostic difference between depth of myometrial invasion and the tumor-free distance from the uterine serosa in endometrial cancer? Gynecol Oncol. 2003;91(3):547-51.
16. Schwab KV, O'Malley DM, Fowler JM, Copeland LJ, Cohn DE. Prospective evaluation of prognostic significance of the tumor-free distance from uterine serosa in surgically staged endometrial adenocarcinoma. Gynecol Oncol. 2009;112(1):146-9.
17. Ozbilen O, Sakarya DK, Bezircioglu I, Kasap B, Yetimalar H, Yigit S. Comparison of myometrial invasion and tumor free distance from uterine serosa in endometrial cancer. Asian Pac J Cancer Prev. 2015;16(2):519-22.
18. Singh N, Hirschowitz L, Zaino R, et al. Pathologic prognostic factors in endometrial carcinoma (other than tumor type and grade). Int J Gynecol Pathol. 2019;38(Suppl 1):S93-S113.

19. De Vitis LA, Schivardi G, Caruso G, et al. Clinicopathological characteristics of multiple-classifier endometrial cancers: a cohort study and systematic review. Int J Gynecol Cancer. 2024;34:229-38.
20. Vergote I, Matias-Guiu X. et al. New FIGO 2023 endometrial cancer staging validation. Welcome to the first molecular classifiers and new pathological variables. Eur J Cancer. 2023 Nov:193:113318. doi: 10.1016/j.ejca.2023.113318.
21. Schwameis R, et al. Verification of the prognostic precision of the new 2023 FIGO staging system in endometrial cancer patients: an international pooled analysis of three ESGO accredited centres. Eur J Cancer. 2023 Nov:193:113317. doi: 10.1016/j.ejca.2023.113317. Epub 2023 Sep 1.
22. Stålberg K, Bjurberg M, Borgfeldt C, Carlson J, Dahm-Kähler P, Flöter-Rådestad A, et al. Lymphovascular space invasion as a predictive factor for lymph node metastases and survival in endometrioid endometrial cancer: a Swedish Gynecologic Cancer Group (SweGCG) study. Acta Oncol. 2019; 58(11):1628-33. doi: 10.1080/0284186X.2019.1643036. Epub 2019 Aug 2. PMID: 31373248.
23. Zannoni GF, Santoro A, Arciuolo D, Travaglino A, Angelico G, Bragantini E, et al. Endometrial cancer and 2023 FIGO staging system: not too soon, but maybe too much? Gynecol Oncol. 2024;189:98-100. doi: 10.1016/j.ygyno.2024.07.678. Epub 2024 Jul 27. PMID: 39068740.
24. Peters EEM, Nucci MR, Gilks CB, McCluggage WG, Bosse T. Histopathology. 2024. https://doi.org/10.1111/his.15272.
25. Peters EEM, Bartosch C, McCluggage WG, Genestie C, Lax SF, Nout R, et al. Reproducibility of lymphovascular space invasion (LVSI) assessment in endometrial cancer. Histopathology. 2019;75(1):128-36. doi: 10.1111/his.13871. Epub 2019 Jun 10. PMID: 31155736; PMCID: PMC6852322.
26. Peters EEM, León-Castillo A, Smit VTHBM, Boennelycke M, Hogdall E, Hogdall C, et al. Defining substantial lymphovascular space invasion in endometrial cancer. Int J Gynecol Pathol. 2022;41(3):220-6. doi: 10.1097/PGP.0000000000000806. Epub 2021 Jul 13. PMID: 34261899.
27. Bosse T, Peters EE, Creutzberg CL, Jürgenliemk-Schulz IM, Jobsen JJ, Mens JW, et al. Substantial lymph-vascular space invasion (LVSI) is a significant risk factor for recurrence in endometrial cancer: a pooled analysis of PORTEC 1 and 2 trials. Eur J Cancer. 2015;51(13):1742-50. doi: 10.1016/j.ejca.2015.05.015. Epub 2015 Jun 3. PMID: 26049688.
28. Dagher C, Bjerre Trent P, Alwaqfi R, Davidson B, Ellenson L, Zhou QC, et al. Oncologic outcomes based on lymphovascular space invasion in node-negative FIGO 2009 stage I endometrioid endometrial adenocarcinoma: a multicenter retrospective cohort study. Int J Gynecol Cancer. 2024; ijgc-2024-005746. doi: 10.1136/ijgc-2024-005746. Epub ahead of print. PMID: 39074932.
29. Bhatnagar AR, Ghanem AI, Alkamachi B, Allo G, Lin CH, Hijaz M, et al. The prognostic impact of substantial lymphovascular space invasion in women with node negative FIGO stage I uterine carcinoma. Gynecol Oncol. 2024;188:44-51. doi: 10.1016/j.ygyno.2024.06.009. Epub 2024 Jun 26. PMID: 38936280.
30. NCCN Guidelines version 3. Endometrial carcinoma, 2024.
31. Rodolakis A, Scambia G, Planchamp F, et al. ESGO/ESHRE/ESGE Guidelines for the fertility-sparing treatment of patients with endometrial carcinoma. Int J Gynecol Cancer. 2023;33:208-23.

32. Mueller JJ, Pedra Nobre S, Braxton K, Alektiar KM, Leitao MM Jr, Aghajanian C, et al. Incidence of pelvic lymph node metastasis using modern FIGO staging and sentinel lymph node mapping with ultrastaging in surgically staged patients with endometrioid and serous endometrial carcinoma. Gynecol Oncol. 2020;157(3):619-23. doi: 10.1016/j.ygyno.2020.03.025. Epub 2020 Apr 1. PMID: 32247604; PMCID: PMC7293586.
33. International Collaboration on Cancer Reporting (iccr-cancer.org). 2021; Version 4.1.
34. Xu Y, Zhao M, Zhang L, Wang T, Wang B, Xue Y, et al. Outcomes of fertility preservation treatments in patients with endometrial cancer with different molecular classifications based on an NGS panel. Front Oncol. 2023;13:1282356. doi: 10.3389/fonc.2023.1282356. PMID: 38023131; PMCID: PMC10665890.
35. Dobrzycka B, Terlikowska KM, Kowalczuk O, Niklinski J, Kinalski M, Terlikowski SJ. Prognosis of Stage I Endometrial Cancer According to the FIGO 2023 Classification Taking into Account Molecular Changes. Cancers (Basel). 2024;16(2):390. doi: 10.3390/cancers16020390. PMID: 38254879; PMCID: PMC10813919.
36. Concin N, Matias-Guiu X, Vergote I, et al. ESGO/ESTRO/ESP guidelines for the management of patients with endometrial carcinoma. Int J Gynecol Cancer. 2021;31:12-39.
37. Rios-Doria E, Abu-Rustum NR, Alektiar KM, et al. Prognosis of isolated tumor cells and use of molecular classification in early stage endometrioid endometrial cancer. Int J Gynecol Cancer. 2024;34:1373-81.
38. Luzarraga Aznar A, Bebia V, Cabrera S. Correspondence on 'Predicting the risk of nodal disease with histological and molecular features in endometrial cancer: the prospective PROME trial' by Bogani et al. Int J Gynecol Cancer. Published Online First: 07 September 2024. doi: 10.1136/ijgc-2024-005958.

7

CHAPTER

Screening for Endometrial Cancer

Geetha Balsarkar

Endometrial cancer develops from cells that line the innermost layer of uterus called endometrial glands. Endometrial cancer is the most common gynecologic malignancy. It is the fourth most common cancer in women in the United States after breast, lung, and colorectal cancers.[1]

Etiologically, endometrial carcinoma usually results from unopposed estrogen stimulation of the endometrium, although non-estrogen-related forms occur as well. The most common presentation of endometrial cancer is postmenopausal bleeding.[2]

Abnormal vaginal bleeding at any age after 35 years is the common symptom of endometrial cancer. Endometrial cancer does not always cause noticeable symptoms, especially in early stages. Some symptoms may be vague, such as abdominal pain or pressure. These nonspecific symptoms can make early detection challenging.

The incidence of EC has been estimated to 1.3–3.05 per 1,000 screened postmenopausal asymptomatic women, the most significant ultrasonographic feature being the thickened endometrium.

There is no standard screening test for endometrial cancer, but there are some guidelines for women at risk or with symptoms:

- *Postmenopausal women:* The American Cancer Society recommends that all women older than 65 years be informed of the risks and symptoms of endometrial cancer and advised to seek evaluation if symptoms occur. There is no evidence to support endometrial cancer screening in asymptomatic women. Evaluation of a patient with suspected disease should include a pregnancy test in women of childbearing age, complete blood count, and prothrombin time and partial thromboplastin time if bleeding is heavy. Most guidelines recommend either transvaginal ultrasonography or endometrial biopsy as the initial study. The mainstay of treatment for endometrial cancer is total hysterectomy with bilateral salpingo-oophorectomy.

- *Women with Lynch syndrome:* Women with or at risk for hereditary non-polyposis colorectal cancer (HNPCC) should be screened annually after age 35.
- *Women with family history:* Asymptomatic women with a first-degree relative diagnosed with endometrial or colorectal cancer before age 60 should be tested.
- *Patients with suspected disease:* A patient with suspected endometrial cancer should have a pregnancy test, complete blood count, and prothrombin time and partial thromboplastin time if bleeding is heavy.

Risk factors for endometrial cancer include:
- Obesity
- Weight gain
- Metabolic syndrome
- Type 2 diabetes
- Hypertension
- Hyperinsulinemia
- Prolonged exposure to unopposed estrogen
- Taking tamoxifen for treatment or prevention of breast cancer.

Women who have a high risk of endometrial cancer may benefit from yearly testing, even without symptoms. Screening helps detect cancer soon after it develops, which may lead to early treatment benefits.[3]

There are two forms of screening for endometrial cancer:
1. *Transvaginal ultrasound:* In a postmenopausal woman without vaginal bleeding, if the endometrium measures >11 mm a biopsy should be considered as the risk of cancer is 6.7%, whereas if the endometrium measures < or = 11 mm a biopsy is not needed as the risk of cancer is extremely low. Transvaginal ultrasound has revealed some limitations, mainly in the group of patients with endometrial thickness between 6 and 14 mm. The absence of endometrial malignancy in women with endometrial thickness < or = 5 mm and the high possibility of cancer in those with endometrial thickness > or = 15 mm has to be taken into account. The use of endometrial thickness as a sole screening test was found not to be of high predictive value and it should be combined with the evaluation of EC risk factors and followed by hysteroscopy and biopsy in suspicious cases. The lack of a universal cut-off value for endometrial thickness makes screening difficult without symptoms.[4]
2. *Endometrial biopsy:* Endometrial biopsy mainly includes Dilation and curettage (D & C), hysteroscopy and hysterectomy. Routine pathological examination of endometrial tissue obtained by any sampling method is the gold standard for the diagnosis of endometrial lesions.

Polyp size on hysteroscopy is a more accurate parameter, because of better sensitivity and specificity. However, while polyp size ≥19.5 mm seems to have a great accuracy for predicting premalignancy and malignancy, histologic evaluation is still necessary to exclude premalignant and malignant polyps.

Tests and procedures used to diagnose endometrial cancer include:

- *Examining the pelvis:* A pelvic examination checks the reproductive organs.
- *Imaging tests:* Pelvic sonography, MRI more accurate than CT scan
- Hysteroscopy-guided endometrial biopsy
- Biopsy by curettage
- Performing surgery to remove tissue like polyp or growth for testing.

At what age should one start screening for endometrial cancer? There is no evidence, however, to support the screening of asymptomatic women and some evidence against screening. Women with or at risk for HNPCC should be offered screening annually by age 35.

The risks of endometrial cancer screening tests include the following:

- Finding endometrial cancer may not improve health or help a woman live longer.
- Some cancers never cause symptoms or become life-threatening, but if found by a screening test, the cancer may be treated.
- False-negative test results can occur. Screening test results may appear to be normal even though endometrial cancer is present.
- False-positive test results can occur. Screening test results may appear to be abnormal even though no cancer is present. A false-positive test result (one that shows there is cancer when there really is not) can cause anxiety and is usually followed by more tests (such as biopsy), which also have risks.
- Side effects may be caused by the test itself.

Side effects that may be caused by screening tests for endometrial cancer include discomfort, bleeding, infection, perforation of the uterus (rare).

We do not yet know exactly what causes most cases of endometrial cancer, but we do know there are risk factors, like obesity and hormone imbalance, that are strongly linked to this cancer. We know that most endometrial cancer cells have estrogen and/or progesterone receptors on their surfaces.

Future of endometrial cancer screening: There is no screening test for endometrial cancer right now. The results of a Mayo Clinic-led study published in Gynecologic Oncology in 2023, however, may help healthcare professionals detect endometrial cancer earlier by testing vaginal fluid for the presence of cancer-specific methylated DNA markers.[5]

REFERENCES

1. Cabrera S, de la Calle I, Baulies S, Gil-Moreno A, Colas E. Screening strategies to improve early diagnosis in endometrial cancer. J Clin Med. 2024;13(18):5445. doi: 10.3390/jcm13185445. PMID: 39336931; PMCID: PMC11432712.
2. Cavkaytar S, Kokanali MK, Ceran U, Topcu HO, Sirvan L, Doganay M. Roles of sonography and hysteroscopy in the detection of premalignant and malignant polyps in women presenting with postmenopausal bleeding and thickened endometrium. Asian Pac J Cancer Prev. 2014;15(13):5355-8. doi: 10.7314/apjcp.2014.15.13.5355. PMID: 25041001.
3. Godoy CE Jr, Antunes A Jr, Morais SS, Pinto-Neto AM, Costa-Paiva L. Accuracy of sonography and hysteroscopy in the diagnosis of premalignant and malignant polyps in postmenopausal women. Rev Bras Ginecol Obstet. 2013;35(6):243-8. doi: 10.1590/s0100-72032013000600002. PMID: 23929196.
4. Tsikouras P, Bacha M, Zervoudis S, Koukouli Z, Iatrakis G, Galazios G, et al. Controversies on transvaginal ultrasound screening for endometrial cancer in asymptomatic postmenopausal women. Rev Med Chir Soc Med Nat Iasi. 2016;120(4):855-60. PMID: 30141611.
5. Zhao X, Yang Y, Fu Y, Lv W, Xu D. DNA methylation detection is a significant biomarker for screening endometrial cancer in premenopausal women with abnormal uterine bleeding. Int J Gynecol Cancer. 2024;34(8):1165-71. doi: 10.1136/ijgc-2024-005723. PMID: 39043572.

8

CHAPTER

Lynch Syndrome

Mala Srivastava, Saloni Chadha

INTRODUCTION

Colorectal cancer is the third most common malignancy worldwide, accounting for approximately 10% of all cancer diagnoses, and it is the second leading cause of cancer-related mortality. In 2020, global estimates indicated over 1.9 million new cases and more than 930,000 deaths due to colorectal cancer. Projections show that by 2040, the incidence will rise to 3.2 million new cases annually (a 63% increase), with related mortality reaching 1.6 million deaths per year (a 73% increase). While the majority of colorectal cancer cases are sporadic, around 5–10% arise from inherited genetic mutations, predominantly associated with Lynch syndrome (hereditary nonpolyposis colorectal cancer, HNPCC). Lynch syndrome carries an elevated lifetime risk of colorectal cancer (up to 80%) and a 60% risk for endometrial cancer. Additionally, it predisposes individuals to other cancers, including gastric, ovarian, small bowel, urothelial (ureter, renal pelvis, bladder), prostate, biliary tract, pancreatic, adrenocortical, brain (glioblastoma), as well as sebaceous gland adenomas and keratoacanthomas.[1] Patients with Lynch syndrome typically develop carcinomas at a younger age compared to the general population, with an average age of onset around 44 years.[2]

PATHOPHYSIOLOGY

Lynch syndrome is an autosomal dominant hereditary disorder caused by pathogenic mutations in key DNA mismatch repair (*MMR*) genes, which are essential for maintaining genomic stability. The key mismatch repair genes involved in Lynch syndrome are *MLH1* (located on chromosome 3p22.2), *MSH2* (chromosome 2p21-16), *MSH6* (chromosome 2p16.3), and *PMS2* (chromosome 7p22.1). Normally, *MLH1* forms a dimer with *PMS2*, creating the MutLα complex, which coordinates the binding of additional proteins involved in mismatch repair, such as DNA helicase, RPA, and DNA polymerases. Similarly, *MSH2* pairs with *MSH6* to identify DNA mismatches via a sliding clamp model, scanning for replication errors. Mutations in these genes impair the formation and function of these protein complexes, leading to an inability to correct DNA replication errors. The accumulation of these mismatches results in microsatellite instability (MSI), most commonly affecting dinucleotide repeats of cytosine and adenine, and promotes the development of malignancies characteristic of Lynch syndrome, including colorectal and extracolonic cancers.[3]

Lifetime cancer risk by specific genes:[4]

- *Any Lynch-related cancer:* Highest risk is for those with the *MSH2* gene mutation (around 80% for both males and females), while those with PMS2 have the lowest risk (around 40% for females and 57% for males).
- *Colorectal cancer:* Highest risk for males with MLH1 or MSH2 mutations (around 55–56%), while the lowest risk is for females with PMS2 mutations (8.5%).
- *Endometrial cancer:* Women with MSH2 or MSH6 mutations have the highest risk (about 44–46%), while those with PMS2 mutations have a lower risk (21%).
- *Gastric cancer:* The highest risk is for males with MLH1 mutations (8.9%) and MSH2 mutations (8.3%), while those with MSH6 or PMS2 mutations have a much lower risk.
- *Ovarian cancer:* Women with MSH2 mutations have the highest risk (13.4%), while those with PMS2 mutations have the lowest (2.5%).
- *Ureter/kidney cancer:* Those with MSH2 mutations face the highest risk (up to 19.5% for females), while the risk is very low for those with PMS2 mutations.
- *Bladder cancer:* Males with MSH2 mutations have the highest risk (13.1%), while the lowest risk is seen in those with MSH6 mutations.
- *Prostate cancer:* Men with MSH2 mutations have the highest risk (24%), while those with PMS2 mutations have the lowest (3.3%).
- *Breast cancer:* Women with MSH6 and MSH2 mutations face the highest risk (around 15%).
- *Brain cancer:* Higher risk in males with MSH2 mutations (6.6%), while those with PMS2 mutations have a very low risk.
- *Small bowel cancer:* Males with MLH1 or MSH2 mutations have the highest risk (around 7–8%), while the risk is lower for those with PMS2 or MSH6 mutations.
- *Pancreatic cancer:* The risk is relatively low across all gene mutations, with the highest being in MLH1 carriers (around 3.7%).
- *Bile duct/gallbladder cancer:* The risk is also low, with the highest risk in MLH1 carriers (4%).

SYMPTOMS

Colorectal cancer is often asymptomatic in its early stages, making routine screening crucial for early detection and timely intervention. When present, symptoms may include alterations in bowel habits, such as persistent diarrhea, constipation, or a narrowing of stool caliber. Hematochezia or melena, indicative of rectal bleeding, may be observed as bright red blood or dark, tarry stools. Patients may experience persistent abdominal discomfort, including cramping, pain, or bloating that does not resolve. Unexplained and sudden weight loss, despite an unchanged diet or lifestyle, can also be a presenting feature. Additionally, chronic occult gastrointestinal bleeding may lead to iron deficiency anemia, manifesting fatigue, weakness, and pallor. These clinical signs warrant further investigation to rule out or confirm colorectal malignancy.[5]

EVALUATION

A detailed personal or family history is essential for identifying individuals at risk for Lynch syndrome. It is diagnosed in individuals with a germline mutation in one of the mismatch repair (*MMR*) genes (*MLH1, MSH2, MSH6, PMS2*) or the *EPCAM* gene, detected through genetic testing. Candidates for germline testing are identified based on clinical criteria, such as the Amsterdam Criteria or Bethesda Guidelines, or via tumor analysis using immunohistochemistry (IHC) or microsatellite instability (MSI) testing.

The *Amsterdam II criteria* are used to identify families at risk for Lynch syndrome (hereditary nonpolyposis colorectal cancer, HNPCC). To meet these criteria, all of the following conditions must be fulfilled:[6]

1. Three or more family members with cancers associated with HNPCC, with at least one being a first-degree relative of the other two.
2. Involvement of two successive generations affected by HNPCC-related cancers.
3. One or more of these cancers diagnosed before the age of 50 years.
4. Familial adenomatous polyposis (FAP) has been excluded as a potential cause.

The *Revised Bethesda Guidelines* are used to determine candidates for Lynch syndrome testing based on specific clinical criteria. It includes the following:[7]

1. Colorectal cancer diagnosed before age 50.
2. Presence of synchronous or metachronous colorectal or other Lynch syndrome-related tumors, regardless of the patient's age.
3. Colorectal cancer exhibiting microsatellite instability or associated with histologic features such as tumor-infiltrating lymphocytes, Crohn-like lymphocytic reaction, mucinous or signet-ring differentiation, or a medullary growth pattern.
4. Colorectal cancer in a patient with one or more first-degree relatives with a Lynch syndrome-related cancer, where at least one cancer was diagnosed before age 50.

5. Colorectal cancer in a patient with two or more first- or second-degree relatives with Lynch syndrome-related cancers, regardless of their ages.

Additionally, clinical prediction models have been developed to estimate the likelihood of an *MMR* gene mutation, aiding in the decision to pursue genetic testing for Lynch syndrome. The *MMRpredict model* evaluates factors such as age at CRC diagnosis, tumor location, and family history of CRC and endometrial cancer, showing high sensitivity (94%) and specificity (91%) in predicting mutations in *MLH1, MSH2, or MSH6*. The *MMRpro model* incorporates personal and family cancer history, along with tumor testing results, to assess the probability of deleterious mutations and future cancer risk, outperforming Bethesda guidelines in discrimination. The *PREMM5 model* estimates mutation risk in MLH1, MSH2/EPCAM, MSH6, and PMS2 based on similar variables and recommends genetic evaluation for scores of 2.5% or higher. Comparative studies reveal that while both MMRpredict and PREMM5 accurately identify MLH1 and MSH2 carriers, MMRpredict shows superior performance for PMS2 mutations, with an area under the curve (AUC) of 0.72 compared to PREMM5's 0.51.[8]

SCREENING IN LYNCH SYNDROME PATIENTS

Screening for Lynch syndrome is essential for the early detection and management of associated cancers, given the high lifetime risk of malignancies such as colorectal and endometrial cancers. Regular surveillance is tailored to the patient's specific risk profile and family history. For colorectal cancer, patients are typically advised to start screening with colonoscopy at an earlier age than the general population, often by age 20–25, or 2–5 years before the age at which the youngest family member was diagnosed with colorectal cancer. Colonoscopies are recommended every 1 to 2 years thereafter to monitor for any early signs of cancer or precancerous lesions.

In addition to colorectal cancer screening, women with Lynch syndrome are advised to undergo endometrial cancer surveillance. This may include annual gynecological examinations and endometrial biopsy starting at age 30–35. For those at high risk of ovarian cancer, prophylactic salpingo-oophorectomy may be considered, and some guidelines suggest ultrasound or serum CA-125 testing, although these methods are less effective in early detection compared to prophylactic surgery.

Regular screening and preventive measures are crucial for managing Lynch syndrome and improving outcomes for affected individuals.[9]

TREATMENT

Surgical intervention remains the primary treatment approach for Lynch syndrome-associated colorectal cancer. Options typically include partial colectomy or total colectomy with ileorectal anastomosis. Given the high risk of subsequent colorectal cancer following partial colectomy and the comparable quality-of-life outcomes between the two procedures, total colectomy is often preferred, particularly for younger patients.

The use of 5-fluorouracil-based adjuvant chemotherapy in Lynch syndrome-related colorectal tumors, especially those in stages I and II, remains a subject of debate regarding its clinical benefit. In contrast, anti-PD-1 antibody therapy has emerged as a highly effective treatment for advanced colorectal cancer with high microsatellite instability (MSI-H). Checkpoint blockade with anti-PD-1 therapy is now considered the preferred first-line treatment for such cases.[10]

REFERENCES

1. Bhattacharya P, Leslie SW, McHugh TW. Lynch Syndrome (Hereditary Nonpolyposis Colorectal Cancer) [Updated 2024 Jun 8]. In: StatPearls [Internet]. Treasure Island (FL): StatPearls Publishing; 2024. Available from: https://www.ncbi.nlm.nih.gov/books/NBK431096/.
2. Lynch HT, de la Chapelle A. Hereditary colorectal cancer. N Engl J Med. 2003;348(10):919-32. DOI: 10.1056/NEJMra012242.
3. Tamura K, Kaneda M, Futagawa M, Takeshita M, Kim S, Nakama M, et al. Genetic and genomic basis of the mismatch repair system involved in Lynch syndrome. Int J Clin Oncol. 2019;24(9):999–1011. doi:10.1007/s10147-019-01494-y. PMID 31273487. S2CID 195795805.
4. Dominguez-Valentin M, Sampson JR, Seppälä TT, et al. Cancer risks by gene, age, and gender in 6350 carriers of pathogenic mismatch repair variants: findings from the prospective Lynch syndrome. Database Genet Med. 2020; 22:15.
5. Dominguez-Valentin M, Haupt S, Seppälä TT, et al. Mortality by age, gene and gender in carriers of pathogenic mismatch repair gene variants receiving surveillance for early cancer diagnosis and treatment: a report from the prospective Lynch syndrome database. EClinicalMedicine. 2023;58: 101909.
6. Menon G, Carr S, Kasi A. Familial Adenomatous Polyposis. 2024 May 5. In: StatPearls [Internet]. Treasure Island (FL): StatPearls Publishing; 2024 Jan. PMID: 30855821.
7. Umar A, Boland CR, Terdiman JP, Syngal S, de la Chapelle A, Rüschoff J, et al. Revised Bethesda Guidelines for hereditary nonpolyposis colorectal cancer (Lynch syndrome) and microsatellite instability. J Natl Cancer Inst. 2004;96(4):261-8. doi: 10.1093/jnci/djh034. PMID: 14970275; PMCID: PMC2933058.
8. Goverde A, Spaander MCW, Nieboer D, van den Ouweland AMW, Dinjens WNM, Dubbink HJ, et al. Evaluation of current prediction models for Lynch syndrome: updating the PREMM5 model to identify PMS2 mutation carriers. Fam Cancer. 2018;17(3):361-70. doi: 10.1007/s10689-017-0039-1. PMID: 28933000; PMCID: PMC5999171.

9. Gupta S, Provenzale D, Llor X, Halverson AL, Grady W, Chung DC, et al. NCCN Guidelines Insights: Genetic/Familial High-risk Assessment: Colorectal, Version 2.2019. J Natl Compr Canc Netw. 2019;17(9):1032–41. doi: 10.6004/jnccn.2016.0108.
10. Stjepanovic N, Moreira L, Carneiro F, Balaguer F, Cervantes A, Balmaña J, et al. ESMO Guidelines Committee. Hereditary gastrointestinal cancers: ESMO Clinical Practice Guidelines for Diagnosis, Treatment and Follow-up. Ann Oncol. 2019;30(10):1558-71. doi: 10.1093/annonc/mdz233.

9 CHAPTER

Radical Hysterectomy: The Wertheim's Surgery

Samar Gupte

INTRODUCTION AND HISTORY

A radical hysterectomy (Wertheim's Surgery) is done to remove the uterus, cervix, upper vagina along with the parametrium, paracervical, and paravaginal tissues primarily described for operable cervical cancer.

Soranus of Ephesus (1st/2nd century AD) a Greek physician[1] described vaginal hysterectomy for the first time. Avenzoar (1091–1162) described a type of uterus removal, whereas in 1507, Giacomo Berengario da Carpi (1460–1530) performed a partial hysterectomy in a case of prolapse.[1] Conrad Langenbeck (1776–1851) performed the first successful hysterectomy in 1813 for endometrial carcinoma. Charles Clay (1801–1893) popularized abdominal hysterectomy in Europe.[1] Wilhelm Alexander Freund (1833–1917) described abdominal removal of a cancerous uterus in 1871.[1]

John Clark (Johns Hopkins at Baltimore) and Emil Ries (Chicago) described radical hysterectomy for the first time in 1895 after discovering cervical cancer in the tissues and lymph nodes beyond the excision limits of the standard hysterectomy.

It was on November 16, 1898, that Ernst Wertheim (1864–1920), an Austrian gynecologist, performed the first radical abdominal hysterectomy (RAH) for cervical cancer **(Fig. 1)**. He published 500 cases done between 1898 and 1911. The principle of Wertheim's hysterectomy was to remove the uterus and the cervix with appropriate parametrium and tissues surrounding the upper vagina and pelvic lymph nodes.[1] His name became eponymous with RAH. In 1901, Friedrich Schauta (1849–1919) described the radical vaginal hysterectomy and reported a lower operative mortality rate than the abdominal approach. Wertheim and Schauta disagreed over whether the abdominal approach was better or the vaginal.[1]

Due to the existing higher mortality and emergence of radiotherapy, RAH was briefly given up as a treatment for cervical cancer.[1] However, it was Joe Vincent Meigs (1892–1963) who modified and repopularized the procedure in the 1950s, adding more extensive pelvic lymphadenectomy. Meigs published a series of 344 cases in 1945. It is this Wertheim-Meigs surgery

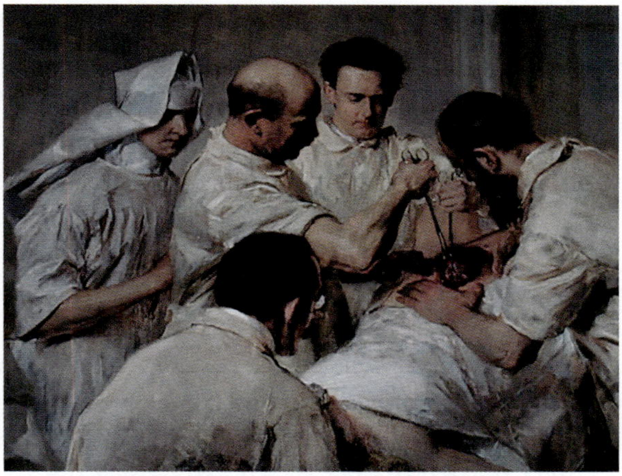

Fig. 1: Ernst Wertheim painted by John Quincy Adams.[1]

that we perform in principle even today. Many others including Okabayashi, Parsons, Ulfelder, Green, Takayama, etc. have made significant contributions to the development of radical hysterectomy as a definitive procedure. Interestingly, over the last 100 years and more, there have been 3 Nobel prize winners and even one nominee during the research and evolution of treatment of cervical cancers.

INDICATIONS

There was a meta-analysis of randomized trials, in the early 2000s, that demonstrated the superiority of radiotherapy and concomitant chemotherapy without surgical removal of the uterus in the treatment of advanced cervical cancer with external radiotherapy.[2]

Thus, current international guidelines recommend avoiding radical hysterectomy in patients with advanced cervical cancer, and instead, referral for definitive chemoradiotherapy is advised.[3]

The indications for a radical hysterectomy can be categorized according to disease.[4]

For cervical cancer:

- Stage 1A1 with lymphovascular space invasion
- Stage 1A2–1B2
- Stage 1B3 (selected)
- Stage IIA1 (selected)

For vaginal cancer: Stage I–II (limited to upper one-third of vagina, usually involving posterior vaginal fornix)

For endometrial cancer: Stage II with gross cervical invasion

Persistent or recurrent cervical cancer after radiotherapy with disease limited to the cervix.

Women with bulky stage IB disease (currently classified as FIGO stage IB3) have been treated with either radical hysterectomy and bilateral pelvic lymphadenectomy or primary radiation therapy, with equivalent survival. However, in most IB3 cases, there is a very high risk of lymph node metastasis, close resection margins, or deep stromal invasion with LVSI, for which adjuvant radiation will be recommended.[4]

PROCEDURE

The extent of hysterectomy required also varies according to the disease. For instance, in early-stage cervical cancer (IA1 or even IA2), a less radical hysterectomy (RH) may be sufficient. In order to standardize these types of hysterectomies, a number of classifications were described. Chief amongst them were the 1974 Piver Rutledge classification and the currently used Querleu-Morrow classification of 2008 which is based on stable anatomic landmarks and also looks at nerve sparing vs. non-nerve sparing radical hysterectomy **(Table 1)**.[5]

TABLE 1: Types of hysterectomy.[5]

	Simple extrafascial hysterectomy	*Modified radical hysterectomy*	*Radical hysterectomy*
Piver and Rutledge classification	Type I	Type II	Type III
Querleu and Morrow classification	Type A	Type B	Type C
Indication	Stage IAI	Type IA1 with LVSI. IA2	Stage IB1 and 1B2, selected Stage IIA
Uterus and cervix	Removed	Removed	Removed
Ovaries	Optional removal	Optional removal	Optional removal
Vaginal margin	None	1–2 cm	Upper one-quarter to one-third
Ureters	Not mobilized	Tunnel through broad ligament	Tunnel through broad ligament
Cardinal ligaments	Divided at uterine and cervical border	Divided where ureter transits broad ligaments	Divided at pelvic side wall
Uterosacral ligaments	Divided at cervical border	Partially removed	Divided near sacral origin
Urinary bladder	Mobilized to base of bladder	Mobilized to upper vagina	Mobilized to middle vagina
Rectum	Not mobilized	Mobilized below cervix	Mobilized below cervix
Surgical approach	Laparotomy or laparoscopy or robotic surgery	Laparotomy or laparoscopy or robotic surgery	Laparotomy or laparoscopy or robotic surgery

To put briefly, Type A is a limited RH that includes removal of cervix to the level of the vaginal fornix, including a paracervical margin. Type B RH (modified RH) includes Type B1 (ureter is unroofed and mobilized laterally) and Type B2 (includes removal of the pelvic lymph nodes). Type C RH includes Type C1 (nerve-sparing resection) and Type C2 (non-nerve sparing). Type D, involves ultra-radical resection of structures lateral to the paracervix and includes Type D1 (dissection to the pelvic sidewall) and Type D2 (resection of the fascia and adjacent musculature).[4]

Patient is usually in a supine or low lithotomy position under general or regional anesthesia (as the case may be). Classically, a radical abdominal hysterectomy is performed via a laparotomy with a mid-line vertical incision, Pfannenstiel, Cherney, or Maylard incision.

Intraoperatively the abdomen is inspected for metastasis. The retroperitoneum is opened, and iliac vessels and ureters are identified. This is followed by a bilateral pelvic lymphadenectomy. Then the paravesical and pararectal spaces are developed and ureters dissected of the peritoneum and traced right up to the ureteric tunnels. The uterine vessels are divided at their origins and lifted medially. The bladder is pushed inferiorly, and the ureteric tunnels are deroofed, allowing the bladder to be dissected further inferiorly to expose the upper vagina anteriorly and laterally. Similarly, the rectum is dissected inferiorly to expose the posterior vaginal wall. The cardinal ligaments, uterosacral ligaments can then be divided as laterally as required to include as much parametrium, paracervical and paravaginal tissues as needed. The vagina is divided at the desired level to complete the radical hysterectomy. Vagina is closed with absorbable sutures.

The immediate complications include bleeding, ureteric, bladder or rectal injuries. Radical hysterectomy has the potential to denervate the pelvic viscera resulting in bladder hypotonia or hypertonia. Somatic nerve damage is occasionally known to occur. The obturator nerve is most commonly damaged during lymphadenectomy. Other nerves like femoral, iliohypogastric, ilioinguinal, genitofemoral, sciatic and peroneal are also vulnerable to damage. Bladder and/or ureteric ischemia leading to fistulae are known to occur but is rare in the absence of prior pelvic radiation. Similarly neuropathic rectal dysfunction may occur, but the incidence is far less as compared to bladder dysfunction. Deep vein thrombosis and its sequelae, infection, lymphoedema and lymphocele formation are some of the other complications.

In younger women with squamous cancers, ovaries can be preserved by ovarian transposition, especially if there is a reasonable chance that postoperative radiation may be needed. The ovaries along with their infundibulopelvic pedicles are fixed outside the pelvis via a subperitoneal tunnel. The site is at least 1.5 cm cephalad to the iliac crest and to the lateral abdominal wall

THE WAY FORWARD

Sentinel lymph node biopsy has also been evaluated in cervical cancer surgery. The benefits of SLN mapping and biopsy include improved detection of microscopic disease and reduction of the side effects of full lymphadenectomy. Nerve-sparing surgery and fertility-preserving options are now being more closely evaluated and pursued.

A large number of retrospective series have demonstrated the feasibility of minimal access surgery for radical hysterectomy. The short-term benefits have been immense. However, recent randomized trials have shown that for early-stage cervical cancer, laparoscopy or robotic surgery to remove the uterus is detrimental compared with laparotomy, resulting in higher mortality rates and more loco-regional relapses.[6] Further prospective randomized trials will be needed to establish the safety and oncological efficacy of minimal access approach for radical hysterectomy.

Treatment of cervical cancer and radical hysterectomy is an example of evolution of surgical oncology, wherein the initial focus was on how effectively the tumor could be removed as the primary treatment. However, in course of time, considering the risks of treatment and recurrence and the development of complementary treatments, there came a balance between treatment efficiency and impact on patient's quality of life. Nevertheless, like in most solid organ tumors, surgery will continue to be a defining factor in the treatment of cervical cancers.

REFERENCES

1. Drouin E, Classe JM, Hautecoeur P. 125 years of Wertheim operation. What next? J of Med and Life. 2023;16:341-3. 10.25122/jml-2022-0082.
2. Green JA, Kirwan JM, Tierney JF, Symonds P, et al. Survival and recurrence after concomitant chemotherapy and radiotherapy for cancer of the uterine cervix: a systematic review and meta-analysis. Lancet. 2001;358(9284):781-6. doi: 10.1016/S0140-6736(01)05965-7.
3. Cibula D, Pötter R, Planchamp F, Avall-Lundqvist E, et al. The European Society of Gynaecological Oncology/European Society for Radiotherapy and Oncology/ European Society of Pathology guidelines for the management of patients with cervical cancer. Radiother Oncol. 2018;127(3):404-16. doi: 10.1016/j.radonc. 2018.03.003.
4. Handa VL, Van Le L. Te Linde's Operative Gynecology, 12 edn. Lippincott Williams & Wilkins, a Wolters Kluwer Business; 2020.
5. Bhatla N, Daisuke A, Sharma DN, Sankaranarayanan R. Cancer of the cervix uteri. Int J Gynecol Obstet. 2018;143 (Suppl. 2):22-36.
6. Ramirez PT, Frumovitz M, Pareja R, Lopez A, et al. Minimally invasive versus abdominal radical hysterectomy for cervical cancer. N Engl J Med. 2018;379(20): 1895-904. doi: 10.1056/NEJMoa180639

4

SECTION

Cervical Cancer: Prevent the Preventable

10. Pathophysiology of Cervical Cancer with FIGO Staging
Anju Singh, Neerja Bhatla

11. FOGSI-GCPR for Cervical Cancer Prevention and Management
Priya Ganesh Kumar

12. Adenocarcinoma of Cervix: An Emerging Issue
Usha Saraiya

13. Radical Trachelectomy
Harshad Parasnis

10

CHAPTER

Pathophysiology of Cervical Cancer with FIGO Staging

Anju Singh, Neerja Bhatla

Cervical cancer is the fourth most common cancer worldwide. According to GLOBOCAN-2022, an estimated 663,301 women were diagnosed with cervical cancer worldwide and about 348,874 women died from disease.[1] India contributes approximately one-fifth of the global burden of cervical cancer, with an estimated 127,526 new cases and 79,906 deaths every year.

Persistent infection with high-risk human papillomavirus (Hr-HPV) is the necessary cause for development of cervical preinvasive and invasive lesions. Other risk factors include early marriage, young age at first intercourse, multiparity, multiple sexual partners, low socioeconomic status, smoking, immunocompromised state, etc. The increased chances of developing cervical cancer in the presence of various risk factors is summarized in **Table 1**. HPV is a double-stranded circular DNA virus that infects skin or mucosal cells. The virus has two main components comprising of a protein cover and double-stranded DNA-containing genetic material within. The double-stranded genome encodes for 6 early proteins (E1, E2, E4, E5, E6, and E7) and 2 late proteins (L1 and L2). The early proteins are responsible for

TABLE 1: Association of various risk factors with the development of cervical cancer.

Risk factor	*Increased risk of cervical cancer*
Young age at first intercourse (<18 years)	2 times
Multiparity as compared to nulliparity: • 3 or 4 births • 7 or more births	 • 2.6 times • 3.8 times
Multiple sexual partners: • 2 partners • 6 or more partners	 • 2 times • 3 times
Current smokers compared to non-smokers	2–3 times
Long-term use of oral contraceptive pills (if >5 years)	1.9 times
HSV-2 coinfection with HPV	3 times

virus replication and the late proteins are the viral structural proteins. Around 130 genotypes of HPV have been identified. The virus types are species and tissue specific. Based on oncogenic potential, they are classified into low-risk and high-risk (oncogenic) types. About 15 of them are attributed to cause cervical cancer. Dr Harald Zur Hausen received the Nobel Prize in Medicine in 2008 for isolating oncogenic HPV strains and elucidating the oncogenic process.

Hr-HPV 16 and 18 are responsible for 65–85% of cases with the global average being about 70%. Other high-risk types include types 31, 33, 35, 39, 45, 51, 52, 56, 58, 59, 68, 73, and 82. In India, the proportion of HPV 16 and 18 is nearly 85%. This virus most commonly spreads through sexual contact which can be either genitalia-to-genitalia, skin-to-skin, or skin-to-genitalia contact. Nonsexual routes of transmission include vertical transmission at the time of childbirth from mother to newborn and by fomites.

HPV enters through small breaks in the cervical epithelium near the squamocolumnar junction and infects the cells of the basal layer. It exists in the episomal form. During the process of oncogenesis, at the cellular level, viral DNA integrates into the host DNA and produces oncoproteins E6 and E7. Oncoprotein E6 binds to tumor suppressor protein P53 and its degradation leads to inhibition of apoptosis and accumulation of DNA damage. E7 proteins bind to retinoblastoma protein pRb and its overexpression results in cell proliferation. Thus, these oncoproteins disrupt the normal regulatory mechanisms of cell division and initiate the process of carcinogenesis.

There is a long period of latency between HPV infection and development of preinvasive and invasive lesions. The majority of infections are clear within 2 years by the body's natural innate immunity. Several risk factors are linked to an increased probability of HPV exposure, such as multiple sexual partners (of self or of the partner) and sexual intercourse at a young age. Multiple births increase the risk of exposure and persistence in the transformation zone. Reproductive tract infections, especially infection with gonorrhea, chlamydia and herpes simplex virus (HSV) 2 have been implicated in persistence and oncogenesis. Others, such as tobacco use or HIV, play a role in immune suppression possibly prompting cervical carcinogenesis. Transplant recipients receiving immunosuppression are also at increased risk for the same reason. It is postulated that suppressed immune function results in a decreased ability to clear HPV, leading to persistent infection and increased risk of developing cervical intraepithelial neoplasia (CIN). Persistent HPV infection of cervix typically develops into CIN and invasive cancer over 10–15 years. Thus, the unique relationship between HPV exposure, prolonged infection, and diminished immune response sets the stage for cervical carcinogenesis.

Preinvasive lesions, i.e., CIN are confined to the basement membrane and are graded based on extent of involvement of thickness of squamous epithelium as follows:

- *CIN 1 (previously termed mild dysplasia):* Dysplastic cells are limited to the lower one-third of the epithelium.
- *CIN 2 (previously termed moderate dysplasia):* Dysplasia involves lower two-thirds of the epithelium.
- *CIN 3 (previously termed severe dysplasia or carcinoma in situ):* Dysplasia affects the full thickness of the epithelium but has not invaded the basement membrane.

The malignant potential of CIN 2+ lesions is much more than CIN 1 lesions. Precancerous lesions arising from the columnar epithelium are referred to as adenocarcinoma in situ (AIS).

These premalignant lesions may remain asymptomatic for years and can be detected using various screening tests [conventional Pap smear, liquid-based cytology, visual inspection with acetic acid (VIA) and, more recently, the HPV test]. The majority of premalignant lesions can be treated on an outpatient basis by ablative or excisional methods. The incidence of cervical cancer below the age of 30 years is low. Therefore, the World Health Organization (WHO) recommends routine screening for cervical cancer is recommended for all women after 30 years of age so that preinvasive lesions can be timely detected, managed and lead to elimination of cervical cancer.

Management of cervical cancer is based on the stage at the time of diagnostic evaluation which is assigned in accordance with the 2018 revised FIGO staging **(Table 2)**. Now, 2018 revised FIGO staging has replaced the older 2009 staging which was mainly based on clinical examination and had major drawback of inability to assess/incorporation of lymph node involvement. The revised version has advantage of incorporation of imaging and pathological findings along with clinical findings, leading to more accurate assessment of locoregional, lymph nodes and distant metastasis. It is also useful for better treatment planning, prognostication and follow-up.[2]

The key changes in the revised 2018 staging are summarized as below:[3]

a. *For Stage IA (micro-invasive) disease:* It considers only depth of invasion. Lateral extent is no longer taken into consideration.
b. *For Stage IB*: An additional substage has been added with cut-off at 2 cm.
c. *For Stage III:* Stage IIIC has been added which includes lymph node metastasis irrespective of tumor size and extension. For lymph node assessment, radiological and pathological findings can be taken into consideration with specific mention with “r” or “p” notation.

TABLE 2: 2018 FIGO Revised staging of carcinoma cervix.

Stage I	The carcinoma is strictly confined to the cervix (extension to the corpus should be disregarded)
IA	Invasive carcinoma that can be diagnosed only by microscopy with a maximum depth of invasion ≤5 mm[a]
IA1	Measured stromal invasion ≤3 mm in depth
IA2	Measured stromal invasion >3 mm and ≤5 mm in depth
IB	Invasive carcinoma with measured deepest invasion >5 mm (greater than Stage IA); lesion limited to the cervix uteri with size measured by maximum tumor diameter[b]
IB1	Invasive carcinoma >5 mm depth of stromal invasion and ≤2 cm in greatest dimension
IB2	Invasive carcinoma >2 cm and ≤4 cm in greatest dimension
IB3	Invasive carcinoma >4 cm in greatest dimension
Stage II	The cervical carcinoma invades beyond the uterus, but has not extended onto the lower third of the vagina or to the pelvic wall
IIA	Involvement limited to the upper two-thirds of the vagina without parametrial invasion
IIA1	Invasive carcinoma ≤4 cm in greatest dimension
IIA2	Invasive carcinoma >4 cm in greatest dimension
IIB	With parametrial invasion but not up to the pelvic wall
Stage III	The carcinoma involves the lower third of the vagina and/or extends to the pelvic wall and/or causes hydronephrosis or non-functioning kidney and/or involves pelvic and/or para-aortic lymph nodes
IIIA	Carcinoma involves the lower third of the vagina, with no extension to the pelvic wall
IIIB	Extension to the pelvic wall and/or hydronephrosis or non-functioning kidney (unless known to be due to another cause)
IIIC	Involvement of pelvic and/or para-aortic lymph nodes (including micro-metastases),[c] irrespective of tumor size and extent (with *r* and *p* notations)
IIIC1	Pelvic lymph node metastasis only
IIIC2	Para-aortic lymph node metastasis
Stage IV	The carcinoma has extended beyond the true pelvis or has involved (biopsy proven) the mucosa of the bladder or rectum. A bullous edema, as such, does not permit a case to be allotted to Stage IV
IVA	Spread of the growth to adjacent organs
IVB	Spread to distant organs

[a] Imaging and pathology can be used to supplement clinical findings.
[b] Vascular/lymphatic space involvement does not change the staging.
[c] Isolated tumor cells do not change the stage.
[r] Imaging
[p] Pathology

Thus, the revised staging provides more precise assessment of disease involvement and spread. It is crucial for treatment planning and reflects survival outcomes more accurately than the previous staging system.[4]

CONCLUSION

Cervical cancer is a public health problem with a well-elucidated pathophysiology with HPV infection being the necessary cause of cervical cancer. It is preventable due to availability of highly effective primary (HPV vaccination) and secondary (screening and treatment) preventive measures. Utilizing our knowledge of pathophysiology to achieve 90-70-90 targets by 2030 as specified by WHO will help to reach the ultimate goal of cervical cancer elimination.

REFERENCES

1. Bray F, Laversanne M, Sung H, et al. Global cancer statistics 2022: GLOBOCAN estimates of incidence and mortality worldwide for 36 cancers in 185 countries. CA Cancer J Clin. 2022;74(3):229-63. doi: 10.3322/caac.21834. Epub 2024 Apr 4.
2. Bhatla N, Berek JS, Cuello Fredes M, et al. Revised FIGO staging for carcinoma of the cervix uteri. Int J Gynecol Obstet. 2019;145(1):129-35.
3. Berek JS, Matsuo K, Grubbs BH, et al. Multidisciplinary perspectives on newly revised 2018 FIGO staging of cancer of the cervix uteri. J Gynecol Oncol. 2019; 30(2):e40. doi: 10.3802/jgo.2019.30.e40. Epub 2018 Dec 28. PMID: 30740962; PMCID: PMC6393641.
4. FOGSI GCPR on Screening and Treatment of Preinvasive lesions of the cervix and HPV vaccination. [30 Jan 2019.] Available from URL https://www.fogsi.org/fogsi-gcpr-on-screening-mangement-of-cervical-precancerous-lesions/.

11

CHAPTER

FOGSI-GCPR for Cervical Cancer Prevention and Management

Priya Ganesh Kumar

INTRODUCTION

India tops the globe in cervical cancer with one lady losing her life to this deadly disease every 7 minutes. Ironically, WHO has declared this as the most preventable cancers in ladies. Since cervical cancer is preceded by Precancerous stage for several years a good amount of 8–10 years, the art and science of identifying this stage by mass scale screening plays a key role in disease development and progression. Since 1950 Cervical Cytology has been used for cervical cancer screening. This no doubt has seen reduction in Cervical Cancer incidences in various countries like Australia, but has not shown any promising results in India due to various barriers. The barriers foreseen by Apex organization and policy makers like FIGO, WHO, AOGIN for Asia Oceania regions to use cytology as screening methods include lack of trained personnels, lack of trained cytotechnicians, lack of proper infrastructure of follow-up with up with colposcopy and treatment with subsequent call-recall system, lack of awareness in the masses for screening which includes health providers and Government bodies. Barriers encountered in the low-resource settings can be found in the FIGO guidance, Section 8–11.[1]

Hence alternative screening method has been sought, reported and used in the low-resource settings—Visual Inspection with Acetic Acid (VIA) and Visual Inspection with Iodine (VILI) discussed in FIGO Guidance, Sections 8–9. Traditionally, cytology positive cases have to undergo further evaluation increasing the visits of the patient. In contrast with, Single Visit Approach (SVA), single test like VIA provides rapid results and treatment with ablative methods like cryotherapy/thermal ablation is made available for women with abnormal tests at the same visit and only very few have to be referred for further management. This approach is called "Screen and Treat". Evidence shows that a single visit VIA with subsequent treatment with cryotherapy for VIA positive cases can reduce the lifetime risk of cervical cancers by 30%, in women in the age group of 35–45 years.[2]

World Health Organization WHO proposed the following targets to achieve Cervical cancer elimination by 2030:

- *90% of girls fully vaccinated with human papillomavirus (HPV) vaccine by 15 years of age*
- *70% of women screened with HPV test at 35 and 45 years of age and all managed appropriately.*
- *30% reduction in mortality from cervical cancer.*

TRIAD FOR CANCER PREVENTION

- *Primary prevention:* Vaccination
- *Secondary prevention:* Screening with HPV and VIA
- *Tertiary prevention:* Clinical diagnosis of precancerous lesions and its early treatment.

Vaccination

Most effective when given to girls below 15 years of age, two doses six months apart. According to FOGSI, vaccination can be given till age of 45 years.

Screening

WHO/IARC, FIGO, and FOGSI are advocating screening with HPV-DNA every 5 years. It has 100% sensitivity with 99% NPV.

CLINICAL DIAGNOSIS

Colposcopy with guided biopsy remains the Gold standard for detecting Cervical Intraepithelial Neoplasias (Precancer lesions). Once detected, precancerous lesions are treated with OPD-based procedures like cryotherapy, LEEP therapy **(Fig. 1)**.

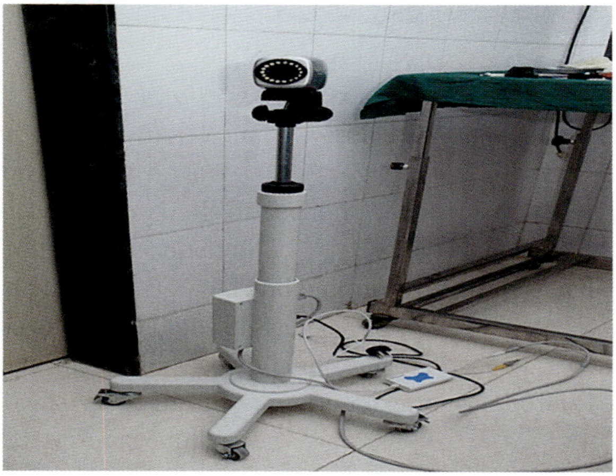

Fig. 1: Colposcope.

DIFFERENT TYPES OF SCREENING METHODS (TABLE 1)

TABLE 1: Different types of screening methods.

Type of screening method	*Sensitivity*	*Specificity*
Cytology Pap Smear	57 (95% CI 38–76%)	93% (95% CI 89–97%)
HPV-DNA	62 % (95% CI 56–63%)	94% (95% CI 92–95%)
VIA In c/o CIN2	79% (95% CI 73–85%)	85 % (95% CI 81–89%)
VIA In c/o CIN3	83% (95% CI 77–89%)	84% (95% CI 80–85%)
VILI	89% (95% CI 83-95%)	84% (95% CI 80–85%)

Source: International Journal of Cancer IJC, Pooled analysis of accuracy of five cervical cancer screening tests assessed in studies in Africa and India.

FOGSI-GCPR

The latest FOGSI-GCPR 2023 was released on 14th April, 2023 at New Delhi MCM of FOGSI **(Fig. 2)**.

VACCINATION

FOGSI-HPV Vaccination Schedule (Table 2)

The following are the different types of vaccine available:

- Bivalent (Cervarix by GSK) licensed for girls 10–45 years
- Quadrivalent (Gardasil by MERCK) licensed for girls 9–45 years and boys 9–26 years

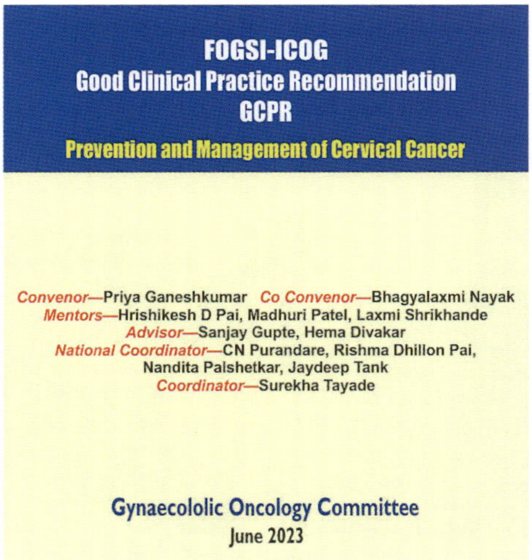

Fig. 2: Latest FOGSI-GCPR 2023.

TABLE 2: Human papillomavirus (HPV) vaccination schedule.

Dose	*Schedule*	*Evidence level and grade of recommendation*
Optimal dose	• Two doses 9–14 years at least 6 months apart • Three doses above 15–26 years (0, 1–2 months, 6 months) • Three doses for older women till 45 years. Regular screening as per guidelines has to be followed in this age group	Level I, Grade A Level II, Grade B
*Reduced dose:** a. Two doses WHO-SAGE recommendation b. Alternative single dose (off-label)	• One or two doses for 9–14 years • One or two doses for 15–20 years • Two doses for 21 years and above • Single dose schedule can be used for girls and boys aged 9–20 years	Level II, Grade B Level II, Grade B
Boys	• *Boys can be vaccinated from 9–26 years:* – 9–14 years 2 doses 0, 6 months – 15–26 years 3 doses 0, 2, 6 months	Level II, Grade C

*Reduced dose schedule of HPV vaccine awaits Drug Controller General of India (DCCI) approval.

- Nonavalent (Gardasil by MERCK) licensed for girls and boys 9–45 years
- Quadrivalent (Cervavac by SIL) licensed for girls and boys 9–26 years[3]

Primary and Secondary Target Groups for Vaccination

- For the prevention of cervical cancer, the WHO-recommended primary target population for HPV vaccination is girls aged 9–14 years before they become sexually active.
- Achieving coverage in girls also reduces the risk of HPV infection for boys.
- Vaccination of secondary target populations, e.g., females aged ≥15 years, boys, older males or men who have sex with men (MSM), is recommended only if this is feasible and affordable, and does not divert resources from the vaccination of the primary target population.

Screening

Visual inspection with acetic acid 3–5%—Once every 3–5 years.

TABLE 3: Interpretation of Visual Inspection with Acetic Acid (VIA) test.

Parameters of aceto white lesion	*VIA positive*	*VIA negative*
Speed of appearance	Appears rapidly and may last for 1–2 minutes	Appears late and quickly disappears (within a minute)
Color intensity	Shiny and cloudy white, more dense, thick and opaque	Pale or dull white, less dense, thin, often translucent
Borders and demarcation	Well demarcated, regular, raised from surrounding epithelium	Patchy with ill-defined, diffuse margins
Location	Restricted to transformation zone mostly, lesions close to or abutting the squamocolumnar junction	Distributed widely in the cervix, not restricted to the transformation zone (TZ)
Color uniformity	Uniformly white	Color intensity varies across the lesion

TABLE 4: HPV-validated test.

HPV-DNA signal amplification	*PCR-based test*	*mRNA-based E6/E7*
Hybrid Capture 2 (HC2; Qiagen, Hilden, Germany)	• Cobase® HPV test (Roche, Pleasanton, USA) • BD Onclarity HPV assay • (Becton Dickinson, Sparks, MD)	Aptima® HPV assay (Hologic, San Diego, CA)
Cervista HPV HR Test (Hologic Inc., Bedford, MA, USA)	• Abbott Real-time High-risk HPV test • PapilloCheck (Greiner Bio-One, Frickenhausen)	
careHPV test (Qiagen Gaithersburg Inc., MD, USA)	• Pretect™ HPV-Proofer (Nor Chip Norway) • Anyplex II HPV HR (Seegene Inc., Seoul, Korea) • Xpert HPV (Cepheid, Sunnyvale, CA, USA)	

Interpretation of VIA Test

See **Table 3**.

Cytology

Conventional pap or with liquid-based cytology (LBC) once every 3 years. LBC is better than conventional pap as it reduces the inflammatory smear report with clean background. Adequacy depends on the cellular count. Conventional pap requires minimum 8000–12,000 cells. LBC requires minimum 5000 cells. LBC has increased sensitivity to detect the LSIL 12% more than conventional pap, whereas for HSIL and cancer, there is no difference in specificity in either LBC or conventional.[4-6]

Human Papillomavirus

It is a highly sensitive test with high NPV value. To be done every 5 years. As per WHO, HPV tests can be done at least twice in a lifetime at 35 and 45 years in low- or middle-income (LMI) countries.

The list of available HPV-validated tests is shown in **Table 4**.

SCREEN AND TREAT WITH PRIMARY HPV SCREENING (FLOWCHART 1)

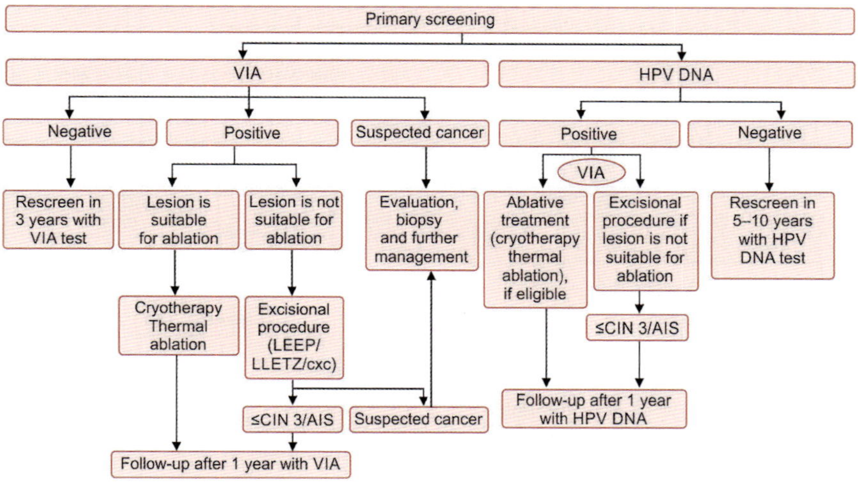

SCREEN, TRIAGE AND TREAT WITH PRIMARY CYTOLOGY (FLOWCHART 2)

Primary cytology screening and colposcopy triage

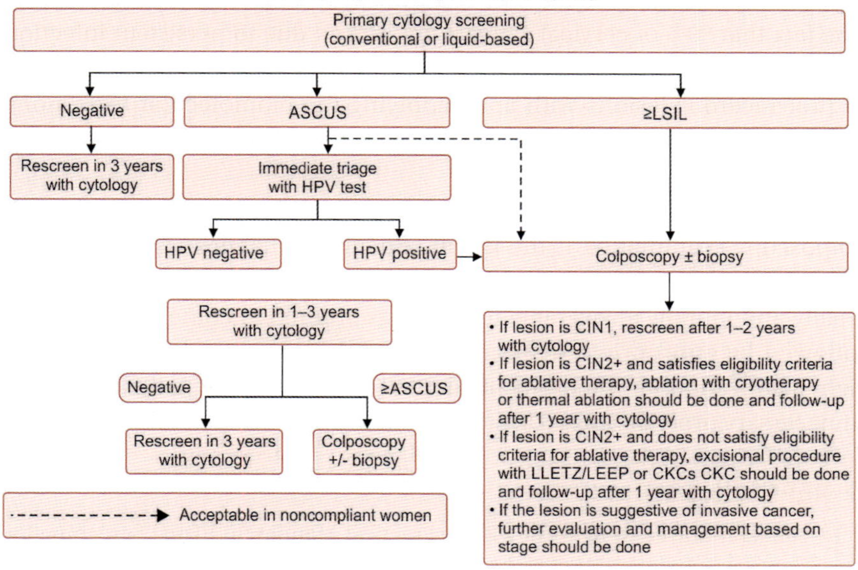

SCREEN, TRIAGE AND TREAT WITH PRIMARY HPV SCREENING (FLOWCHART 3)

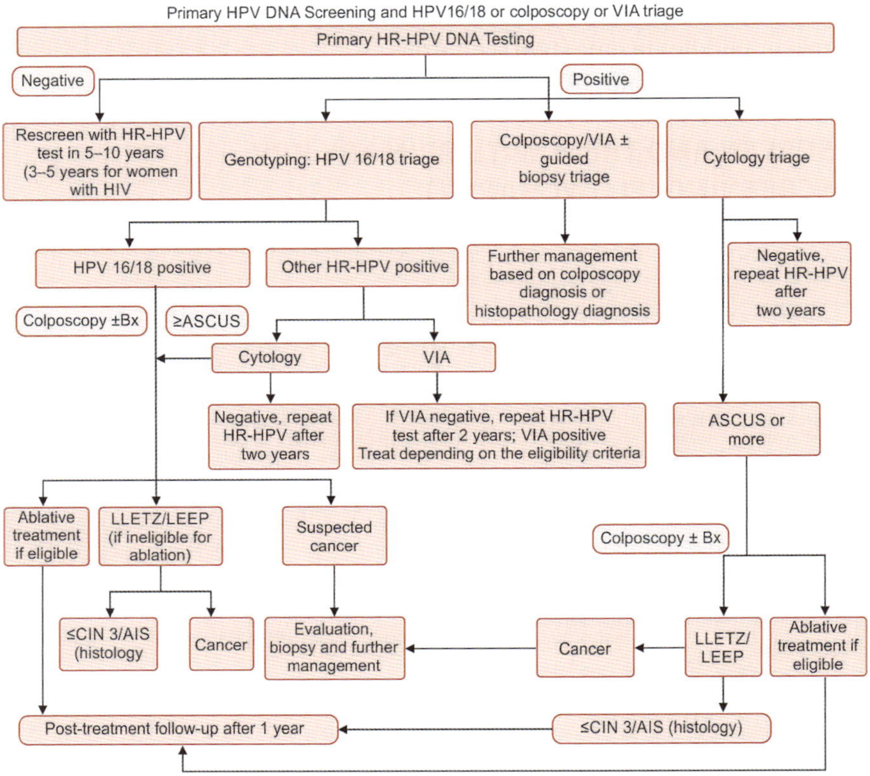

CONCLUSION

The fact that 99% of cervical cancers are caused due to persistent infection with HR-HPV has opened up new vistas in the field of concurrent diagnostics of precancerous lesions with aptly applying the biomolecular tests along with cytology as co-test in Colposcopy detected lesions confirmed on histopathology.[7]

Judicious and scientific application of biomolecular tests along with colposcopy examination is the key in concurrent diagnostics for management of CIN cases. In this, google era with patient always well read, we are legally and morally answerable for the tests ordered to come to a diagnosis followed by appropriate treatment. This helps the clinicians to give the right justification for the protocol adopted for treating the patients. By this, unnecessary procedures and hysterectomies can be avoided.[8]

REFERENCES

1. Sankaranarayanan R, Wesley RS. A Practical Manual on Visual Screening for Cervical Neoplasia: IARC Technical Publication No. 41. Lyon: IARC Press; 2013.

2. Sankaranarayanan R, Basu P, Wesley RS, Mahe C, Keita N, Mbalawa CC, et al. Accuracy of visual screening for cervical neoplasia: Results from an IARC multicentre study in India and Africa. Int J Cancer. 2004;110:907–13.
3. Colposcopy in Practical Gynaecology, 2nd edition; CBS Publications.
4. International Agency for research on Cancer. Handbook of Cancer Prevention: Vol 10: Cervical Screening. Lyon: IARC Press; 2015.
5. Colposcopy terminology: the 2011 IFCPC nomenclature-IARC Publications.
6. iarc.fr Ifcpc.org.2017/10.
7. https://www.fogsi.org/fogsi-gcpr-on-prevention-and-management-of-cervical-cancer-june-2023/.
8. https://www.fogsi.org/fogsi-gcpr-on-prevention-and-management-of-cervical-cancer-june-2024/.

12 CHAPTER

Adenocarcinoma of Cervix: An Emerging Issue

Usha Saraiya

INTRODUCTION

Cervical cancer continues to be a major health issue for women especially in low and low-to-middle income countries of the world.

In 2023, 6,60,6000 women suffered from cervical cancer in the world and 3,50,000 women died of it.[1]

With the introduction of WHO's Cervical Cancer Elimination Initiative launched in 2018, these statistics will hopefully change. With emphasis on screening and proper treatment of precancerous conditions in women from the age of 35–65 and systematic vaccination of all girls between the ages of 9′–26, the situation will come under control.

Bhatla, Meena and Kumari[2] have indicated the progress made in India in 2021. The recent age adjusted rate for India is 17.7 which has significantly come down, since the beginning of this century.

However, some difficult cases will continue to appear and gynecologists have to be well informed and well prepared to look after these cases.

One such condition is the adenocarcinoma of the cervix which has now become an emerging issue. Overall, adenocarcinoma incidence is 6.6 per 1,00,000 women in the age group of 35–65.[3] However, if you consider only the women in the age group of 30–39 it rises to 11.2 per 1,00,000. Hence, it is very essential to study endocervical smears in this age group.

In the last decade, an increase in the incidence of adenocarcinoma of the cervix has been noted. As such all adenocarcinomas seem to show an increase such as endometrial, ovarian and colonic. The rise in endocervical adenocarcinoma may perhaps be due to better control of squamous cell carcinoma which is diagnosed and treated at precancerous stage. It may also be due to the use of dual modalities of screening, i.e., Cytology + HPV testing currently in practice. It also happens that endocervical and squamous carcinoma are coexisting. It is usually HPV-related tumor and can attack both types of epithelia. HPV types associated with it are usually 16 and 18, or 31, 35. That is the primary risk factor for both adenocarcinoma-in-situ and invasive adenocarcinoma.

TABLE 1: Classification of adenocarcinoma cervix.

RCOG (UK)	*WHO (modified)*
Low-grade cervical glandular intraepithelial neoplasia (L-CGIN)	Endocervical glandular dysplasia (EGD)
High-grade cervical glandular intraepithelial neoplasia (H-CGIN)	Adenocarcinoma in situ (AIS)
Endocervical adenocarcinoma	*Adenocarcinomas:* a. HPV-associated and HPV-independent b. Viloglandular c. Endometrioid d. Neuroendocrine e. Glassy cell f. Gastric, clear cell and mesonephric

It is reported by Doorbar[4] that the HPV virus may lie in the latent phase in the crypts of the Endocervix or in the crysts of the tonsils. It surfaces when the individual's immunity goes down and gets activated and forms tumors.

The change from adenocarcinoma-in-situ to invasive phase may take 13 years, same as for squamous. However, diagnostic difficulties are more for adenocarcinoma than for squamous and that may cause some delay in diagnosis.

There are many classifications available for adenocarcinoma cervix. **Table 1** gives the standard ones given by RCOG and by WHO, which are commonly used. Basically, there are three dysplastic categories: In situ and Invasive Lesions. WHO classifies the endocervical carcinoma into several subtypes. Some of the endocervical carcinomas are HPV-independent.[5] This may lead to delay in diagnosis. If atypical glandular cells are found and the patient is HPV negative, further investigations may not get done. Hence it is important to be aware of this condition. Further reference to colposcopy is necessary and a repeat of conventional and liquid based cytology has to recommended.

There is an interesting category called SMILE lesions which include all Stratified Mucin producing Intraepithelial Lesions. These arise from the reserve cells and start in the transformation zone. It is actually a malignant transformation of the metaplastic cells. They are characterized by both glandular and squamous elements and P16 +ve on immune histochemistry and also +ve for mucicarmine.

This was earlier described by Adolf Stafl in 1975 where in he explained how atypical metaplasia as diagnosed on colposcopy is acted upon by some carcinogen. At that time, in 1975, it was not known that HPV is the carcinogen which triggers malignancy. **Flowcharts 1A and B** explain how atypical metaplasia needs to be watched carefully as further progression may lead towards the development of carcinoma.

Flowcharts 1A and B: Graphic representation of possible evolutions of early squamous metaplastic process (from A. Stafl)

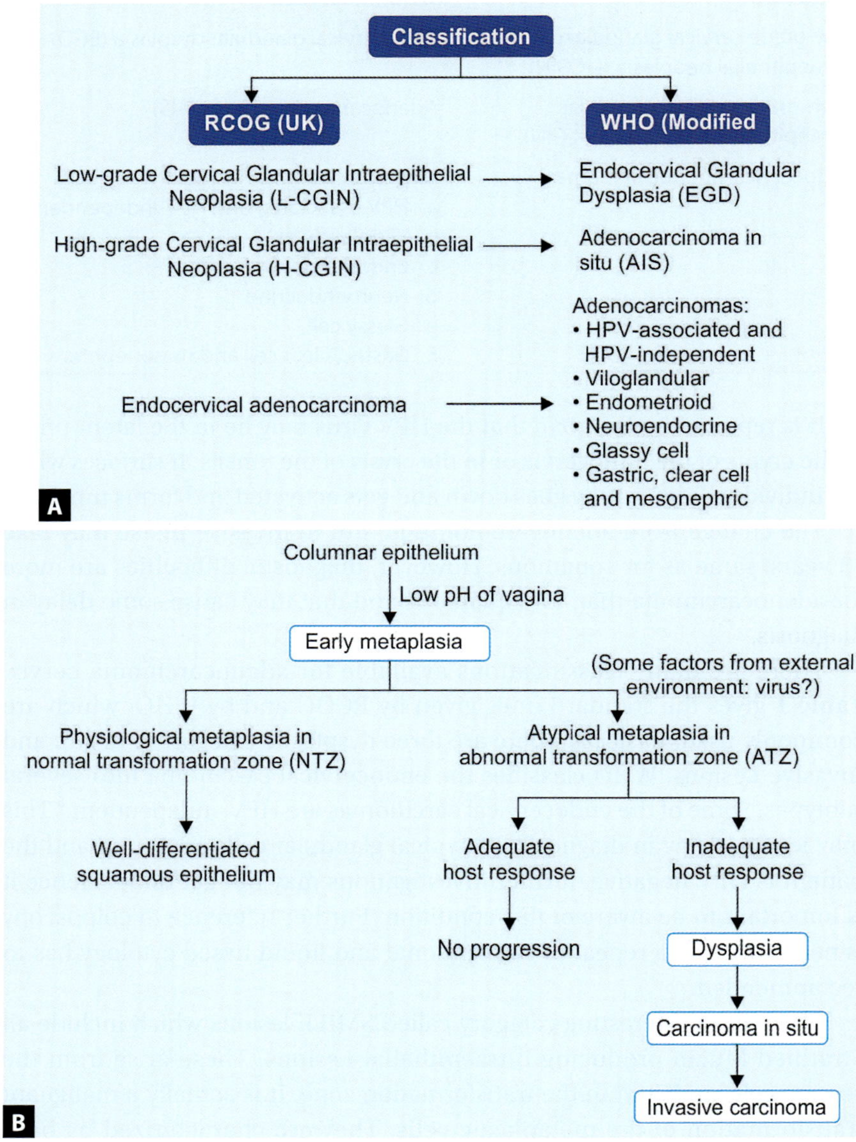

HPV is a multicentric disease[6] and the reactions of the affected tissue can be different. In the endocervix, there are skipped lesions with partial gland involvement **(Figures 1 to 6)**. It may go upwards to the endometrium, or it may grow downwards and cover the ectocervix. The stromal reaction is edema and/or inflammation. There is marked structural complexity of endocervical glands, making it difficult to diagnose invasion or lymphovascular space involvement.

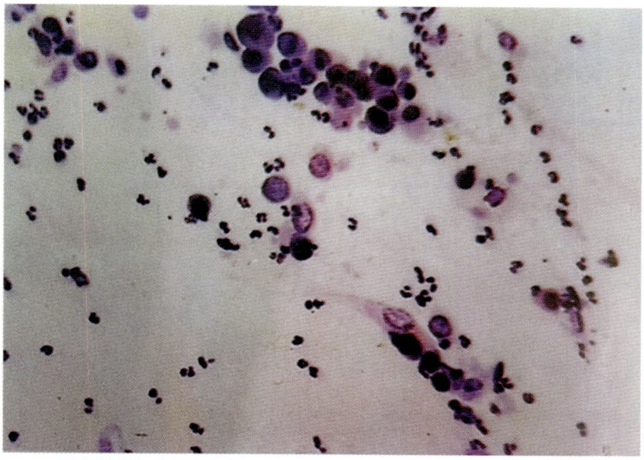

Fig. 1: Adenocarcinoma in situ (AIS) small cells.

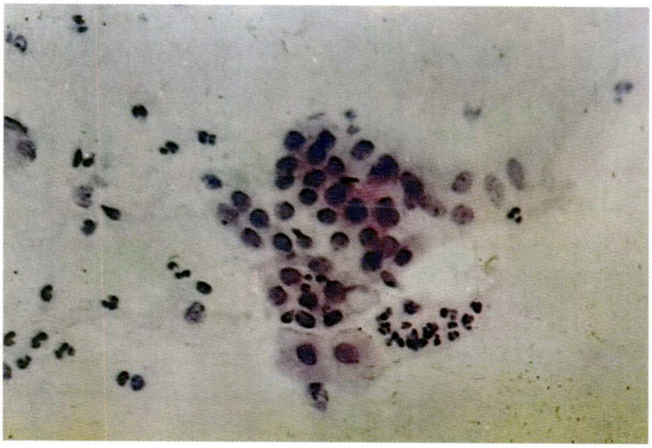

Fig. 2: Atypical glandular cells.

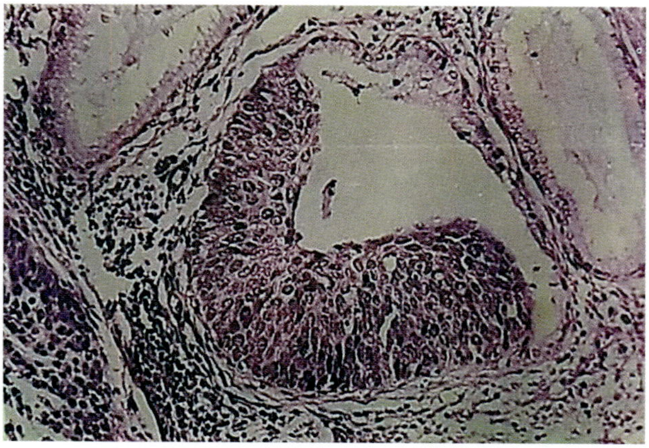

Fig. 3: Part of the crypts has abnormal epithelium.

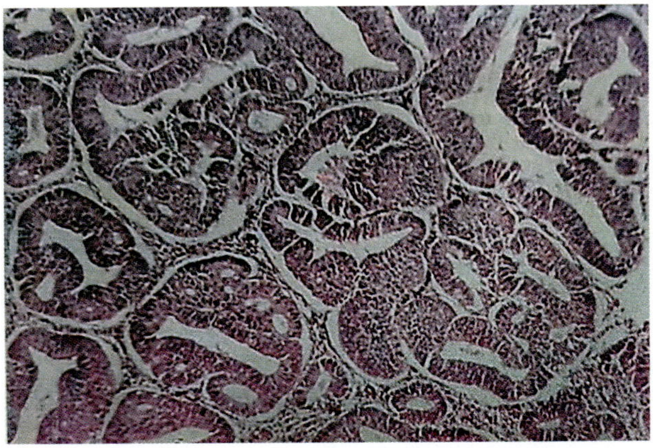

Fig. 4: Adenocarcinoma crypts are closely packed.

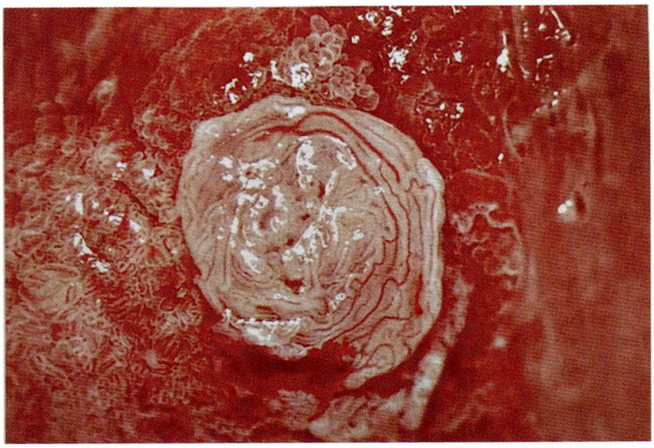

Fig. 5: Elevated papillary Acetowhite lesion with bizarre vessels.

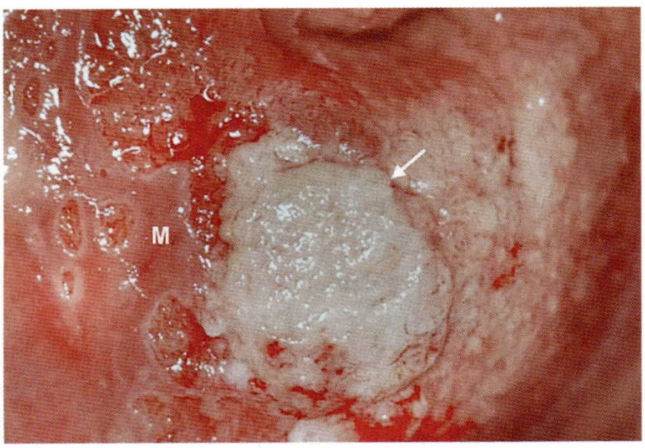

Fig. 6: Excision biopsy and resultant histology revealed adenocarcinoma.

Pradhan, Zaibo[7] have reported on 3000 cases of atypical glandular cells in Pap smears. They recommended that all such cases be investigated by endocervical and endometrial histology.

The use of dual-stained cytology as of great value in the diagnosis in cases of abnormal cytology as it also indicates the presence of HPV infection.[8]

COLPOSCOPY

Colposcopy is a valuable aid to diagnose this condition. The main advantage is that it raises a suspicion that endocervical epithelium is involved. A Colposcopist has to be very vigilant and not miss the warning signs. A good correlation of cytology, colposcopy, and HPV testing is required for a correct diagnosis.

Whenever the Colposcopist sees columnar epithelium on the ectocervix and especially if it makes the cervix look red and "angry" there is some cause for anxiety. The differential diagnosis may be cervicitis, immature atypical squamous metaplasia or recent trauma of delivery or abortion. There may be an Acetowhite area. If there is no rim to that area, it is more significant.

Some conservative treatment may be given, and patient may be called for a review preferably postmenstrual. The entire cervix should be studied before applying acetic acid. Study of the papillae which may be enlarged or fused and should be noted. Gland openings may be cuffed or large and open. There may be variegated red and white patches all over the cervix. The discharge from the endocervix may be milky white or like a profuse mucorrhea. A look into the endocervix may show raised white areas in between the columnar glandular structure. These may be "Skipped" lesions.[9]

If all the above patterns are noted along with abnormal vessels, the suspicion of malignancy is raised. Vessels may be small or big, bizarre-shaped and bleed on touch. Comma-shaped or root-like vessels are noted.

Highly suspicious areas are the yellow or brown areas. Friability and necrotic tissue indicate malignancy. Examine the swab after swabbing the cervix. If it has friable tissue on it, it is a sign of advanced disease.[10]

Prior HPV testing and cytology reports should be available before doing colposcopy. LBC reports are more informative than conventional pap smears or if suspicions are raised on colposcopy, both conventional and liquid-base cytology should be repeated, and HPV test needs to be done.[11]

PRINCIPLES OF MANAGEMENT

Histological diagnosis is the mainstay for planning treatment. The procedure of Cold Knife Conization (CKC) and LLETZ are both diagnostic and therapeutic. WHO[11] recommends CKC as there were fewer recurrences. Specimen needs to check with serial sectioning in view of the possibility of "skipped" lesions. If margins are clear and uninvolved and if LVSI is –ve, then recurrence in unlikely. Immunohistochemistry for P16 and Ki67 is helpful for prognosis. This treatment may be adequate for a young patient desirous of fertility.

If micro- or frank invasion is noted and also if P16 Ki67 are positive further treatment may be done as per FIGO guidelines. For young women desirous of fertility, trachelectomy or ART procedures may be considered. Fertility-sparing onco-surgery is very well developed in India and every young woman should have access to it.[12]

TAKE HOME MESSAGE

- Colposcopy has an important but limited role. The most important is to raise suspicion.
- Investigate and treat the patient thoroughly before planning treatment.
- It may be helpful to have a Gynecological Oncologist in the team.
  - Antibiotics and suppositories to clear infection.
  - Check HPV and HIV status and other blood tests.
  - USG scan or MRI is very useful to have a detailed topography of the endocervix and ectocervix.
  - The immunological status of the patient and also medications given for other diseases have to be reviewed.
  - Inform patients relatives and take proper consent.

What is in the Realm of Research Today will Translate into Clinic Practice Tomorrow?

Research has a far-reaching impact on humanity: Surgery should be scheduled in an operation theater with all facilities available. One should be prepared for hemorrhage. Adequate stromal tissue in the specimen should be taken to exclude invasion. Endocervical curettage may be done and sent separately for biopsy. Packing maybe needed. Patients should be kept under observation for 1 day in hospital and follow up for 15 days with antibiotic cover. Review the case with histology and immunohistochemistry results.

"As is our Pathology,
So is our Practice."

REFERENCES

1. Globocan 2024 https://gco.iarc.fr.
2. Bhatla N, Meena J, Kumari S, Banerjee D, Singh P, Natarajan J. Cervical cancer prevention efforts in India. Indian Gynecol Oncol. 2021;19:41.
3. Miniello G. Immediate Colpsocopy: Vulvoscopy and Anoscopy. Edra SPA. Milano. 2021. pp. 103-10.
4. Doorbar J. Pathogenesis of Papillomaviruses in Humans. In 'Human Emerging and Re-imerging Infections. Viral and Parasitic Infections (Vol 1). In: Singh SK (Ed). John Wiley & Sons, New Jersey, USA. 2016.

5. Conrad RD, Liu AH, Wentzensen N, Zhang RR, Dunn ST, Wang SS, et al. Cytologic patterns of cervical adenocarcinomas with emphasis on factors associated with underdiagnosis. Cancer Cytopathol. 2018;126(11):950-8. https://doi.org/10.1002/cncy.2205
6. Sortey K, Lulla M, Saraiya U. J of Obst and Gyn of India. 1998:48:1.
7. Pradhan D, Li Z. Ocque R, Patadji S, Zhao C. Clinical significance of atypical glandular cells in pap tests: an analysis of more than 3000 cases at a large academic women's center. Cancer Cytopathol. 2016;124:589-95.
8. Luttmer R, Dijkstra MG, Snijders PJF, Berkhof J, van Kemenade FJ, Rozendaal L, et al. p16/Ki-67 dual-stained cytology for detecting cervical (pre) cancer in an HPV-positive gynecologic outpatient population. Mod Pathol. 2016;29:870-8.
9. Miniello G. Easy Colposcopy. Edra SPA Milano, 2019.
10. Saraiya U, Miniello G. Cytology and Colposcopy in Gynaecological Practice. Jaypee Brosthers Medical Publishers. 2009. pp. 179-80.
11. World Health Organization. WHO Guidelines for Screening and Treatment of Precancerous Lesions for Cervical Cancer Prevention. Available at https://www.who.int/reproductivehealth/publications/cancers/screening_and_Treatment_of_ precancerous_lesions
12. Saraiya UB. New Paradigms in Cervical Cancer Prevention. J Obstet Gynecol India. 2024;74:295-302. https://doi.org/10.1007/s13224-024-02050-z

13 CHAPTER

Radical Trachelectomy

Harshad Parasnis

INTRODUCTION

Radical trachelectomy is a fertility preserving surgical procedure used primarily to treat early-stage cervical cancer in women who wish to preserve their fertility. Vaginal radical trachelectomy with laparoscopic pelvic lymphadenectomy was first introduced by Daniel Dargent in 1994.

During radical trachelectomy procedure, the cervix, parametria (surrounding tissue), upper part (1–2 cm) of the vagina and paracolpos are removed, while the uterus remains intact. This allows for the possibility of future pregnancies, although they would typically need to be delivered via the cesarean section.

The procedure is generally considered for women with early-stage cervical cancer who meet specific criteria.[1] Before embarking on this surgery, it is important for patients to discuss the risks and benefits as well as the implications for future pregnancies and potential complications with their gynecologic oncologist as well as healthcare provider.

INDICATIONS

- Women with early-stage cervical cancer who wish to preserve their fertility.
- Early-stage cervical cancer—FIGO stage IA2 or stage IB1 (tumor ≤2 cm)
- No involvement of the upper endocervical canal
- No evidence of lymph node metastasis as determined by magnetic resonance imaging (MRI)/computed tomography (CT)
- No additional abnormal lesions in the vagina (by colposcopy)
- Squamous cell carcinoma or well-differentiated adenocarcinoma
- Cervical cancer recurrence

CONTRAINDICATIONS

- Prior pelvic radiation therapy
- Poorly differentiated adenocarcinoma, small cell carcinoma or neuro-endocrine tumors, papillary serous carcinoma, and sarcomas

TYPES OF SURGICAL TECHNIQUES

- Abdominal approach
- Vaginal approach
- Laparoscopic or robotic-assisted approach

Abdominal or laparoscopic approaches have gained more acceptance than vaginal approach for radical trachelectomy. Since 1994 to date, there have been approximately 1500 radical vaginal trachelectomies reported with decreasing frequency, whereas publications on abdominal or robotic radical trachelectomy have increased.[2]

PREOPERATIVE PREPARATION

- Informed consent, accepting the option of choosing either abdominal radical hysterectomy or abdominal radical trachelectomy
- Patient evaluation and counseling
- Imaging studies (MRI, CT, PET)
- Blood tests and biopsy (HPR)
- Anesthesia fitness

SURGICAL STEPS

Before performing radical trachelectomy, it is important to rule out pelvic lymph node involvement. Pelvic lymphadenectomy, either by laparoscopic or open approach should be performed first to evaluate lymph node involvement. The pelvic lymph node dissection should include external, internal, and common iliac lymph node and obturator lymph nodes.[3] If lymph nodes are involved, then the procedure is abandoned.

Frozen section is important to ascertain that all surgical margins are free of disease ensuring a complete fertility-sparing procedure.

ABDOMINAL APPROACH

- Abdominal incision (horizontal or vertical)
- Exploration of pelvic organs
- Bilateral pelvic lymph node dissection
- Retroperitoneal space opened
- Ureter and bladder dissected and uterine artery transected at origin
- Parametria and paracolpos dissected
- Posterior cul-de-sac incised and uterosacral divided
- Clamps are placed on the lower uterine segment at the level of the internal os followed by transection of the specimen
- Vaginal mucosa is sutured to the remaining cervical stump, followed by a prophylactic cerclage
- Closure of abdominal incision

VAGINAL APPROACH

- Vaginal incision and dissection of 2 cm vaginal cuff
- Dissection of bladder, ureters and parametria
- Opening pouch of Douglas
- Bilateral proximal parametrectomy after identification of the uterine artery
- The cervix is cut 5 mm below the isthmus. The specimen was sent for immediate pathological examination, for checking free endocervical margin. Then the pouch of Douglas was closed, and a permanent cerclage was put at the level of the isthmus.
- Finally, the vaginoisthmic anastomosis was performed.

LAPAROSCOPIC OR ROBOTIC-ASSISTED APPROACH

- Multiple 5-port incisions and insertion of laparoscope or robotic arms
- Dissection of parametria and ureters
- Ligation of uterine arteries
- Removal of cervix, upper vagina, and parametria
- Pelvic lymph node dissection (PLND)
- Reconstruction of vagina
- Cervical cerclage
- Port closure

POSTOPERATIVE CARE

- Hospital stay (2–4 days)
- Pain management
- Antibiotics and anticoagulants
- Monitoring for complications
- Follow-up every 3 months for 2 years, then every 6 months for 3 years, then yearly

Benefits

- Preservation of uterus and fertility
- Reduced risk of cervical cancer recurrence
- Minimally invasive options can be exercised

Risks and Complications

- Infection
- Bleeding
- Infertility or miscarriage
- Preterm labor (rate of preterm delivery appears to be proportional to cervical volume loss)

- Lymphedema
- Nerve damage
- Urinary or bowel dysfunction

Recovery

- Hospital stay (2–4 days)
- Rest and pelvic rest (6–8 weeks)

Fertility Considerations

- Pregnancy success rates vary (50–80%)
- Increased risk of preterm labor and cervical insufficiency
- Cervical cerclage may be recommended

Emotional Considerations

- Anxiety and stress
- Emotional impact on relationships and fertility
- Counseling recommended

Postsurgery Follow-up

- Regular Pap tests
- Colposcopy
- Imaging studies (as needed)
- Consult a gynecologic oncologist or healthcare provider for personalized guidance and treatment options

OUTCOMES AFTER RADICAL TRACHELECTOMY

Oncological outcomes: Radical trachelectomy is oncologically safe. The recurrence rate is around 5% and the mortality rate is around 3%. Patient selection is critical to decrease the risk of recurrence. Risk factors for recurrence include lesions greater than 2 cm, presence of lymph-vascular space invasion, unfavorable histology, and close (defined as <5 mm) surgical margins.

Fertility results: About 15% of women who undergo radical trachelectomy may be infertile, mostly due to cervical stenosis and require further treatment with assisted reproductive technology.[4]

Pregnancy outcomes: The pregnancy rate is around 70% for women who want to conceive. Pregnancy rates following radical vaginal trachelectomy are consistently high at 53–76%. In their reviews, Smith, et al. and Nezhat, et al. concluded that radical vaginal trachelectomy offers the highest pregnancy rates among different radical trachelectomy techniques.

The rate of preterm delivery following radical vaginal trachelectomy is 30–45%. Preterm delivery following radical vaginal trachelectomy is mainly due to shortening of cervical length and cervical incompetence with the attendant increase in the risk of infection and premature rupture of membranes.[5]

REFERENCES

1. Smith ES, Moon AS, O'Hanlon R, et al. Radical trachelectomy for the treatment of early-stage cervical cancer: a systematic review. Obstet Gynecol. 2020;136(3): 533-42.
2. Kohler C, Plaikner A, Siegler K, et al. Radical vaginal trachelectomy: long-term oncologic and fertility outcomes in patients with early cervical cancer. Int J Gynecol Cancer. 2024;34:799-805.
3. Dargent D, Martin X, Sacchetoni A, et al. Laparoscopic vaginal radical trachelectomy. Cancer. 2000;88:1877-82.
4. Cottrell CM, Ohaegbulam GC, Smith JR, et al. Fertility-sparing treatment in cervical cancer: abdominal trachelectomy. Best Pract Res Clin Obstet Gynaecol. 2021;75:72- 81.
5. Nezhat C, Roman RA, Rambhatla A, et al. Reproductive and oncologic outcomes after fertility-sparing surgery for early-stage cervical cancer: a systematic review. Fertil Steril. 2020;113:685-703.

5

SECTION

Vulvar and Vaginal Carcinoma: Untouched Domain

14. **Basics of Vulvar Anatomy with Benign and Malignant Vulvar Diseases**
Niranjan Chavan, Helen Kamei

15. **Various Treatment Modalities of Vulva and Vaginal Diseases**
Bhagyalaxmi Nayak, Monika Dewan

16. **Surgery for Vulvar Cancer**
Kanmani Murugesan, Amita Maheshwari

14

CHAPTER

Basics of Vulvar Anatomy with Benign and Malignant Vulvar Diseases

Niranjan Chavan, Helen Kamei

ANATOMY

The vulva represents the external female genitalia. It includes the mons pubis, labia majora and minora, clitoris, vulvar vestibule, vestibular bulbs, greater (Bartholin's) and lesser vestibular glands, Skene and paraurethral glands and urethral and vaginal orifices. Mons pubis is a pad of fat extending to labia majora, which are prominent folds extending to perineum. Skin over it has hair and subcutaneous layer of tissue. Labia minora are also cutaneous folds but devoid of subcutaneous fat and hair. Vaginal vestibule harbors the openings of the urethra, vagina, and the paired glands—Bartholin, Skene, lesser vestibular glands. The Bartholin glands are lined by columnar epithelium, located at 5 and 7 o'clock connected to the vestibule by 2 cm duct. Clitoris is composed of midline body, distal glans and paired crura. It is lined with thinly stratified squamous epithelium and bears prominent nerve bundles **(Fig. 1)**.

BLOOD SUPPLY, LYMPHATICS, AND INNERVATION (FIG. 2)

The external pudendal artery supplies the skin and subcutaneous tissue of mons. Clitoral arteries are one of the terminal branches of the internal

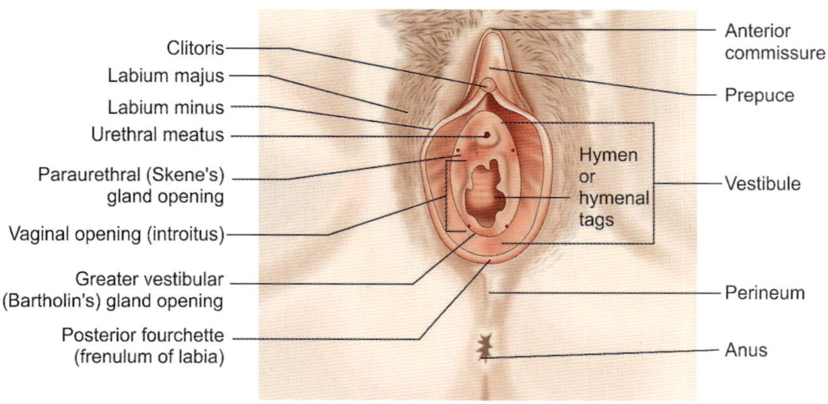

Fig. 1: Vulva.

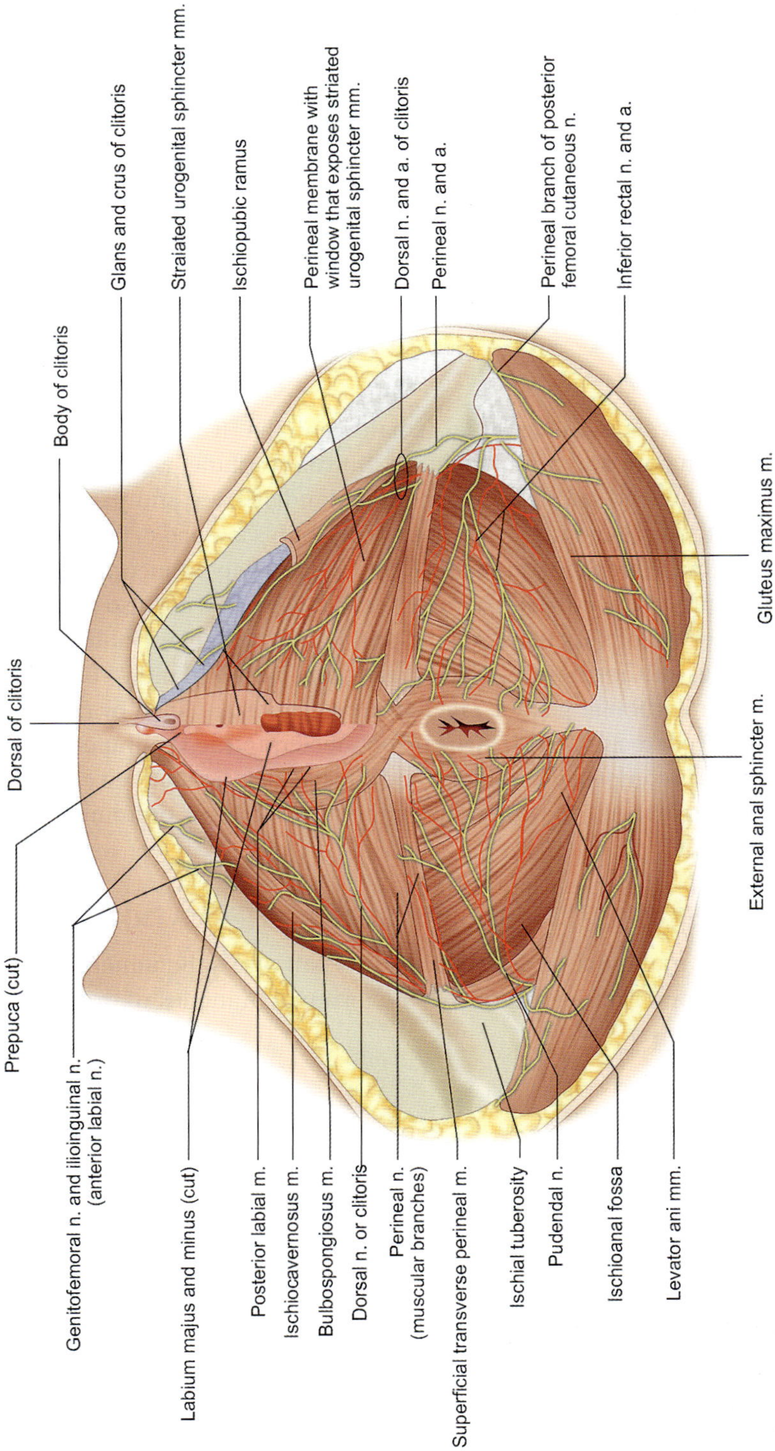

Fig. 2: Blood supply and innervation of vulva.

pudendal artery, which gives off additional branches to the perineum too. Venous drainage has similar course to the arteries except clitoral veins which drain into the internal pudendal veins.

Vulva and perineal lymphatics drain into superficial and deep inguinal nodes. Superficial inguinal nodes are found in the membranous layer of the subcutaneous thigh, superficial to the fascia lata. The deep inguinal nodes are located deep to the fascia lata in the femoral triangle. Efferent channels of the deep inguinal nodes drain into the external iliac nodes. Deep inguinal nodes may also get direct drainage of the glans and corpora cavernosa of the clitoris.

Branches of pudendal nerve provide both sensory and motor innervations. Posterior cutaneous nerve of the thigh provides additional perineal branches.

VULVAR LESIONS: BENIGN AND MALIGNANT

Gynecological visits for vulvar pathology have been increasing and may range from benign to malignant causes. Benign lesions can be treated conservatively or with simple excision unlike premalignant/malignant lesions, which requires a more intensive evaluation, follow-up, and treatment. So, it is imperative that vulvar lesion is differentiated properly from benign to premalignant and malignant as benign lesion may still need biopsy with histopathological evaluation to make a correct diagnosis and exclude malignancy. Vulvar cancer is uncommon compared to other malignancies in terms of incidence and mortality; also, if diagnosed early, it is curable. Also, surgery for vulvar cancer is now more acceptable in terms of morbidity and reconstructive surgery as an adjunct has come a long way in overcoming the deformity both anatomical and functional, associated with radical excision. Radiation as primary or adjuvant treatment for advanced disease helps with keeping the disease in check.

Benign Vulvar Lesions

Benign pathology of vulva may range from cystic or solid or atrophic lesions. Such lesions include Bartholin's cyst/abscess, Gardner's cyst, mucinous cyst, sebaceous cyst, milia, hemangioma, granuloma, lymphangioma, syringoma, schwannoma, endometriosis, leiomyoma, melanosis, hidradenoma, melanocytic naevi, lipoma, lymphangioma, etc.

These lesions may be first seen by gynecologist or dermatologist. The 2011 International Society for the Study of Vulvovaginal Disease (ISSVD) classified vulvar dermatological disorders according to their clinical appearance. This morphological classification combined with history and physical examination helps with identifying the nature of the lesion although in some cases **(Box 1)**.

BOX 1: 2011 International Society for the Study of Vulvovaginal Disease (ISSVD) terminology and classification of vulvar dermatological disorders.

1. *Skin-colored lesions:*
   A. Papules and nodules—epidermal cyst, etc.
   B. Plaques—Liches sclerosus, etc.
2. *Red lesions—patches and plaques:*
   A. Eczematous lesion and lichenified—Paget's disease, etc.
   B. Intact epithelium—candidiasis
3. *Red lesions—papules and nodules:*
   A. Papules—Hidradenitis suppurativa, etc.
   B. Nodules—Furuncles, etc.
4. *White lesions:*
   A. Papules and nodules—Fordyce spots, etc.
   B. Patches and plaques—VIN, etc.
5. *Dark-colored lesions:*
   A. Papules and nodules—Melanoma, etc.
   B. Patches—Lichen planus, etc.
6. *Blisters:*
   A. Vesicles and bullae—Herpes virus infection
   B. Pustules—Folliculitis, etc.
7. *Erosion and ulcers:* Eroded VIN lesion, excoriations, etc.
8. *Edema:*
   A. Skin-colored—postradiation obstruction, etc.
   B. Pink or red-colored—cellulitis, etc.

Biopsy may still be needed to confirm diagnosis and to exclude malignancy. Seborrheic keratosis characterized by proliferation of parabasal cells is usually asymptomatic and affects young women. Condyloma acuminatum presents as warts in sexually active women and associated with low-risk HPV infection (6 and 11). Papillary hidradenoma, well-circumscribed lesion due to branching and interconnecting epithelial and stromal elements. Chondroid syringoma, constituted by epithelial, myoepithelial and stroma, even though benign may rarely have adenocarcinoma arising out of it. Fibroadenoma, a biphasic epithelial-stromal tumor, can recur if incompletely excised. Phyllodes tumor, a rapidly growing biphasic neoplasm, has mammary-like epithelium. Bartholin cysts may be asymptomatic. Secondary infection may present as abscess and painful mass. Bartholin gland hyperplasia, adenoma and adenomyoma are uncommon and usually small solid lesions.

Depending on the type of lesions, treatment may vary from mere observation to medical management to excision. Symptomatic seborrheic keratosis may be treated with cryotherapy/electrosurgery or dermabrasion. Condyloma acuminatum may require excision/cautery or topical imiquimod. Hidradenoma, chondroid syringoma, Bartholin cyst and fibroadenoma may be treated with excision.

Most vulvar lesions are easily identified and managed but premalignant lesions and superimposed malignancy should be borne in mind, wherein lies the importance of detail evaluation and biopsy.

Malignant Vulvar Lesions

Amongst gynecological malignancy, vulvar malignancy is the least common. Patients usually present with vulvar lesion, pruritus and less frequently pain, bleeding, dysuria, dyschezia and sometimes with inguinal lymphadenopathy. Human papilloma virus is associated with majority of vulvar cancer, lichen sclerosus of the vulva is also associated with increased risk. The outcome is better with HPV-associated lesions. Aside from these two associations, other risk factors for vulvar malignancy include age, immunocompromised women, smoking, precancerous lesions of vulva, cancer cervix.

ETIOPATHOLOGY AND TERMINOLOGY

Various histologic subtypes of vulvar cancer include the following:

- *Carcinomas:* Squamous cell carcinoma, adenocarcinoma, Bartholin gland carcinoma, Paget's disease, Merkel cell tumors, verrucous and basal cell carcinoma
- Melanomas
- *Sarcoma:* Leiomyosarcoma, malignant fibrous histiocytoma, epithelial sarcoma, malignant rhabdoid tumor
- Metastatic
- Yolk sac tumor

Precursors lesion referred to as vulvar intraepithelial neoplasia (VIN) or vulvar squamous intraepithelial lesions (SIL) have been noted with disease continuity leading to vulvar malignancy. The College of American Pathology (CAP) and American Society for Colposcopy and Cervical Pathology (ASCCP) tried to clear the perplexing terminology for the precursor lesion through Lower Anogenital Squamous Terminology (LAST) guidelines publication in 2012. A 2-tiered nomenclature: Low-grade squamous intraepithelial lesion (LSIL) and high-grade squamous intraepithelial lesion (HSIL) were used for describing the pathology including cervix, vagina, vulva, anus, perineum, and pelvis. The ISSVD in 2015 categorized the lesion as LSIL, HSIL, and VIN differentiated.

In 2020, the WHO based on molecular data, revised classification of vulvar tumors in relation to human papilloma virus (HPV): HPV-associated and HPV-independent. VIN 1 is categorized under low-grade lesion while VIN 2 and 3 are categorized as high-grade lesion. SIL associated with HPV shows maturation abnormalities, nuclear hyperchromasia, cytological and architectural atypia, elevated mitosis with mitosis in upper epidermal layers and p16 positive. Similarly, the HPV-associated squamous carcinoma is positive for p16 and has infiltrating islands of malignant cells with desmoplastic/inflammatory stroma. Sometime high-grade lesion may be found adjacent to the malignant lesion. SIL-HPV independent is usually associated with chronic inflammatory disease and characteristic finding includes atypia of basal layer with negative p16. Squamous cell carcinoma, HPV-independent, bears well-differentiated keratinizing carcinoma with keratin pearl formation. However, differentiating it from HPV-associated carcinoma by histopathological examination may be difficult; presence of adjacent epithelium bearing features of lichen sclerosus/planus or differentiated VIN may be helpful for diagnosis. Basal cell carcinoma of vulva has similar disease biology as other skin sites. Adenocarcinoma of mammary gland type of vulva pathology is similar to breast carcinoma and locally aggressive disease. Bartholin gland carcinoma requires involvement of anatomical site and compatible histology for diagnosis. Paget disease of the vulva is in-situ adenocarcinoma of vulva. Secondary Paget disease is noted as secondary involvement by carcinoma of the rectum, bladder or cervix. Carcinomas of sweat glands origin and adenocarcinoma of intestinal type usually bear native features descriptive of the tissue histology. Germ cell tumors of vulva usually represent yolk sac tumor.

DIAGNOSTIC EVALUATION

There is no effective screening method for premalignant lesions. Comprehensive history taking with examination is helpful. Biopsy remains the mainstay for diagnosis. The three ring vulvoscopy concept is evolving and helpful for determining not only the disease extent but is useful for evaluation of patient with persistent symptoms despite treatment. The tissue basis for vulvoscopy is like colposcopy except for concentration of acetic acid and duration of application. Biopsy methods can be simple punch biopsy or excision biopsy, or suture assisted. If malignancy is confirmed, metastatic evaluation is essential. Staging of the disease is surgical but imaging may help in planning treatment **(Box 2)**.

Vulvar diseases pose considerable issues for women. While some benign lesions need no treatment, it is important to keep in mind that some vulvar disorders are premalignant and that there may be superimposed malignancy. So, appropriate evaluation should be done for appropriate treatment. Surveillance/follow-up is an important part of management of chronic and premalignant vulvar disorders. Premalignant lesions can be treated with topical Imiquimod, excision or photodynamic/laser therapy. Vulvectomy as surgical treatment has come a long way from debilitating, disfiguring modality to a more conservative, albeit curative for early-stage cancers. Reconstructive surgery complements recovery and quality of life in case of more radical surgery.

BOX 2: FIGO staging of vulva.

Stage	Description
IA	Tumor size ≤2 cm and stromal invasion ≤1 mm*
IB	Tumor size >2 cm or stromal invasion >1 mm*
II	Tumor of any size with extension to lower one-third of the urethra, lower one-third of the vagina, lower one-third of the anus with negative nodes
III	Tumor of any size with extension to upper part of adjacent perineal structures, or with any number of nonfixed, nonulcerated lymph nodes
IIIA	Tumor of any size with disease extension to upper two-thirds of the urethra, upper two-thirds of the vagina, bladder mucosa, rectal mucosa, or regional lymph node metastases ≤5 mm
IIIB	Regional lymph node metastases >5 mm
IIIC	Regional lymph node metastases with extracapsular spread
IV	Tumor of any size fixed to bone, or fixed, ulcerated lymph node metastases, or distant metastases
IVA	Disease fixed to pelvic bone, or fixed or ulcerated regional lymph node metastases
IVB	Distant metastases

SUGGESTED READING

1. Current ISSVD Terminology and Classification of Vulvar Diseases Clinical Diagnosis, updated January 23, 2016.
2. Female genital tumours. WHO Classification of Tumours, 5th edition.
3. Vulvar Lesions: Diagnostic evaluation UpToDate 2024.
4. Williams' Gynecology.

15

CHAPTER

Various Treatment Modalities of Vulva and Vaginal Diseases

Bhagyalaxmi Nayak, Monika Dewan

Vulval cancer is an uncommon malignancy. It represents about 5–8% of gynecological cancer. Squamous cell carcinoma (SCC) accounts for 85–90% of cases. The vulvar SCC can be categorized into human papillomavirus (HPV)-dependent and HPV-independent subtypes based on etiopathogenesis.[1]

Diagnosis-wedge or Keyes punch biopsy, usually in OPD under local anesthesia is sufficient. Imaging provides crucial information on the status of tumor extension to deeper tissues, lymph nodes, and distant organs. Based on magnetic resonance imaging (MRI) findings, around 83% of the vulvar lesions can be accurately classified staged.[2]

STAGING

International federation of gynaecology and obstetrics (FIGO) has introduced the revised 2021 staging for vulvar cancer, emphasizing the role of imaging in the staging of vulvar cancer.[1]

TREATMENT

There is paradigm shift of cancer surgery from radical resection to conservative. It offers the patient a good quality of life without oncological compromise.

Vulval cancer treatment includes management of primary lesion and management of lymph nodes independently.

Management of Early Disease

Primary lesion in early stages is managed by radical excision of vulva with at least 1–2 cm free margin is recommended. Margins can be reduced if the tumor is close to midline structures such as the clitoris, anus, or urethra to preserve their functions. In case of positive margins (<8 mm from the tumor), re-excision or if unresectable or involving the urethra, anus, or vagina, adjuvant external beam radiotherapy is recommended.[3]

Inguinofemoral lymphadenectomy (IFLD) should be done for stages IB or higher. Unilateral lymphadenectomy is ideal when tumor is <4 cm and located ≥2 cm from the midline. For a tumor within 2 cm of the vulvar midline, bilateral IFLD is recommended.

The landmarks for inguino-femoral lymph node dissection (IFLND) incision are anterior superior iliac spine laterally and the pubic tubercle medially. The incision is given 1 cm above the inguinal ligament parallel to it on medial two-thirds of the line joining the above landmarks. Transverse incision or a lazy S incision can give good exposure to the dissection field. Just below the skin lies the fascia Camper which does not house the nodes and hence it is prudent to leave this layer undisturbed to help in wound healing. Minimal handling of skin margins and use of skin hooks gives better wound healing. The lymph nodes lie below this layer beneath the Scarpa's fascia. Enlarged nodes show up themselves and are easy to identify. Nodes are a superficial transverse chain and deep longitudinal chain. Both the groups need to be removed. The deep inguinal nodes lie in the femoral triangle, which is bounded by inguinal ligament superiorly, adductor longus medially and sartorius laterally. The femoral vein, artery and nerve are arranged from the medial to lateral. And as the lymphatic channels lie medial to the femoral vein it is unnecessary to dissect laterally. The lymph node harvest of at least six nodes is considered adequate. The highest node lies in the fossa ovalis and is named as Cloquet's node. This node is sent separately for HP study. Sartorius transposition may be considered in lean women to prevent femoral blow out and also when radiation is anticipated. Placing a vacuum drain for around 10 days or till the collection is significantly reduced could prevent lymphocele formation. Early ambulation and physiotherapy lessen the degree of lymphedema.

Previously, radical surgery with IFLD was considered the gold standard treatment for early-stage vulvar cancer. Although radical surgery improved the 5-year survival rates but there was significant morbidity like infections, pain, lymphocele, and chronic lymphedema responsible for prolonged hospitalization and delay in adjuvant therapy.

Moreover, only 10–26% of the dissected lymph nodes demonstrate metastases. Clinical examination alone is not reliable. Imaging such as ultrasound, computed tomography (CT), MRI, and PET are reported to have a wide sensitivity range (45–86%), and negative likelihood of ratio range (0.12–0.6) and hence are less reliable.

Sentinel lymph node (SLN) biopsy has a sensitivity of 92% and NPV of 97–98% in identifying metastases in comparison to IFLD.[3] Contralateral lymphadenectomy is advised for patients with positive lymph node metastases or undetectable SLN. SNLB in vulva is rapidly becoming the norm for tumors less than 4 cm diameter based on the findings of GROINSS-VI. This study concludes that in patients with negative sentinel node (SLN) it is safe to omit a complete inguinofemoral lymphadenectomy in the treatment of early-stage vulval cancer. The preliminary data from GROINS-VII suggests that radiotherapy is a safer alternative treatment in sentinel node metastasis ≤2 mm and metastases >2 mm should undergo completion IFLND instead of upfront radiotherapy. In case of clinically positive and enlarged inguinal nodes, full IFLND is avoided. Only enlarged nodes are removed, followed by adjuvant therapy. This will prevent complications of dual modalities of treatment (Complete IFLND and RT).

Ulcerated or fixed nodes are treated by primary radiotherapy with or without chemotherapy. However, non-responders may require resection of the node.

Radical Vulvectomy ± Resection of the Distal Urethra or Vagina

This procedure is usually indicated for multifocal disease or lesions involving lower urethra and vagina. The entire vulva and deep tissues ± clitoris, lower urethra and lower vagina are removed with triple incision technique. The vulval incision is elliptical originating from mons pubis anteriorly to perineal area posteriorly along the labiocrural fold to the perineal area. When the lesion involves urethra or vagina, distal 1 cm urethra can be excised without loss of continence. The raw area around the urethra should be left to heal by granulation. Using good diathermy gives a clean field to work due to reduced blood loss. Primary closure may be possible in some cases when the skin around is lax. Vacuum drain is an option. Pressure bandage with dynaplast aids in reducing seroma formation.

Reconstruction of Large Defects

In the majority cases primary closure of the vulval defect is possible due to lax skin. Difficulty arises when there is large tumor with subsequent large defect after surgery in terms of closure. Moreover, when the lesion is at mons, perineal body, or surgery done after radiation therapy, the problem of primary closure becomes challenging. Healing by secondary intention is a possibility with long period of hospitalization and lot of scarring. Some sort of graft or flap is required to overcome this issue. Flaps are recommended in cases at high-risk of breakdown and when cosmetic result is likely to be poor. It is also a treatment of choice in cases of superficial vulvectomy done for VIN or in noninvasive Paget's disease of vulva. Commonly, rotation and transposition flaps are being used with rich blood supply. Lotus petal flap is a variant of rotational and transposition flap, which thrives on blood supply from terminal branches of internal pudendal vessels in perineal area as it is simple and easy to perform with rare breakdown.

Management of Advance Stage Disease

Stage III or IVA should receive radiotherapy with concurrent chemotherapy. Patients with residual tumor managed by resection, or if unresectable, external beam radiotherapy is preferred. Palliative care and better quality of life are the primary treatment goals in patients with distant metastases. However, platinum-based chemotherapy regimens alone or in combination with paclitaxel, vinorelbine, 5-fluorouracil, or mitomycin C are frequently used but further studies are mandatory to make any further recommendations.[2] Gefitinib and trastuzumab combination regimen has shown efficacy by increasing the radiosensitivity of the vulvar lesion though experimental.[3]

The 5-year survival rate is 86%, 53%, and 19% for localized disease, regional spread, and distant spread, respectively.[3]

Patient surveillance should include history and careful clinical examination for vulvar lesions and cervical, perianal, and vaginal neoplasms, all associated with HPV infection.[2] It is essential to emphasize the symptoms of tumor recurrence, including new lesion/mass, vulvar itching, leg or groin pain, lower extremity lymphedema, urinary symptoms, weight loss, and cough. Laboratory studies, imaging, and biopsies are recommended for all suspicious lesions. Given the rarity of primary vulvar cancer, data for treating recurrences are even scarcer and no clear standard of care exists.[3]

Management of Carcinoma Vagina

Primary vaginal cancer is rare, and reported in only 1–2% of all the gynecological cancers.

The primary vaginal cancer diagnosis is by exclusion of involvement of the cervix and/or vulva as well as any malignant lesion arising in the vagina within 5 years after the treatment of cervical cancer.[4]

Vaginal cancer is also strongly associated with the human papillomavirus.

Women usually present with bleeding or a malodorous discharge, pain, and symptoms of disseminated disease depend on the site of metastases.

Diagnosis of vaginal cancer is by biopsy of the lesion and a clinical assessment. Modern imaging techniques such as CT, MRI, and PET are helpful for diagnosis, local staging, and assessment of recurrence and complications.

Vaginal cancer is staged according to the FIGO staging and is primarily based on clinical findings.

The treatment of primary vaginal cancer is complex. Different modalities of treatment can be offered to patients affected by this disease including surgery, radiotherapy, chemotherapy, or a combination of some or all of the above.

SURGERY

The role of surgery is limited and only useful in certain situations, as listed below:

Surgical Management of Stage I Disease (Early Disease)

A. Upper Vaginal Disease

i. Tumor limited to the mucosa in Stage I disease.
ii. If the uterus is in situ, radical hysterectomy, vaginectomy aiming for 1 cm disease-free margins with pelvic lymphadenopathy. If the uterus has been removed, radical vaginectomy with pelvic lymphadenectomy.[5]

B. Lower Vaginal Disease

i. Radical wide local excision with 1 cm margins with bilateral groin node dissection
ii. Ovarian transposition during surgery and pre-radiation especially in young women to prevent the adverse effects of radiation-induced menopause
iii. Central recurrence after radiation treatment
iv. Palliative management of recurrent or advanced diseases, e.g., urinary diversion or colostomy to improve quality of life.

Radiation

In the majority of cases and especially in advanced stages, radiation constitutes the cornerstone of treatment. This is a combination of external beam radiation (EBRT) and intracavitary radiotherapy or brachytherapy (ICRT). The principal advantage of radiation is organ preservation.[4]

Concurrent Chemoradiotherapy

Concurrent chemotherapy and radiation therapy (CCRT) have been employed in treating vaginal cancer from the data extrapolated from locally advanced cervical cancer. A large US National Cancer Data Base (NCDB) study showed that CCRT was an independent prognostic factor for better overall survival (56 months for CCRT vs. 41 months for radiation therapy). Currently, standard of care for locally advanced vaginal cancer is combination of EBRT and brachytherapy to a total dose of 70–80 Gy with concomitant weekly cisplatin-based chemotherapy.[5]

In a larger series of patients with vaginal cancer, the 5-year relative survival was 96%, 64–84%, 53–58%, 36%, and 18–36% for stages O, I, II, III, and IV, respectively.[4] Other factors that negatively impact prognosis include advanced stage, tumor size >4 cm, older age, and possibly tumor location outside of the upper third of the vagina.

The most significant difference that can be made in vaginal and vulval cancer incidence is by highlighting the importance HPV vaccination throughout the world.

REFERENCES

1. Merlo AS. Modern treatment of vulvar cancer. Radiol Oncol. 2020; 54:371-6. doi: 10.2478/raon-2020-0053.
2. Virarkar M, Vulasala SS, Daoud T, Javadi S, Lall C, Bhosale P. Vulvar Cancer: 2021 Revised FIGO Staging System and the Role of Imaging. Cancers (Basel). 2022;14(9):2264. doi: 10.3390/cancers14092264. PMID: 35565394; PMCID: PMC9102312.
3. Abu-Rustum NR, Yashar CM, Rebecca A, et al. Vulvar Cancer, Version 3.2024, NCCN Clinical Practice Guidelines in Oncology. J Natl Compr Canc Netw. 2024;22(2):117-35.
4. Adams TS, Rogers LJ, Cuello MA. Volume 155, Issue S1, Special Issue: FIGO Cancer Report 2021. International Journal of Gynaecology & Obstetrics. 2021 pp. 19-27.
5. Jhingran A. Updates in the treatment of vaginal cancer. International Journal of Gynaecologic Cancer. 2022;32:344-51.

16

CHAPTER

Surgery for Vulvar Cancer

Kanmani Murugesan, Amita Maheshwari

INTRODUCTION

Vulvar cancer is rare, constituting approximately 5% of all gynecologic malignancies. Surgery for vulvar cancer has evolved significantly over the past five decades from radical en bloc resection of primary lesion and groin nodes through a single butterfly incision to a more individualized approach, with the aim to reduce surgical morbidity without compromising the oncological outcomes. While planning surgery, the tumor size, site, involvement of adjacent vital structures, lymph nodal status, histology type, patient's performance status and morbidity anticipated post-surgery should be considered **(Figs. 1 and 2)**.

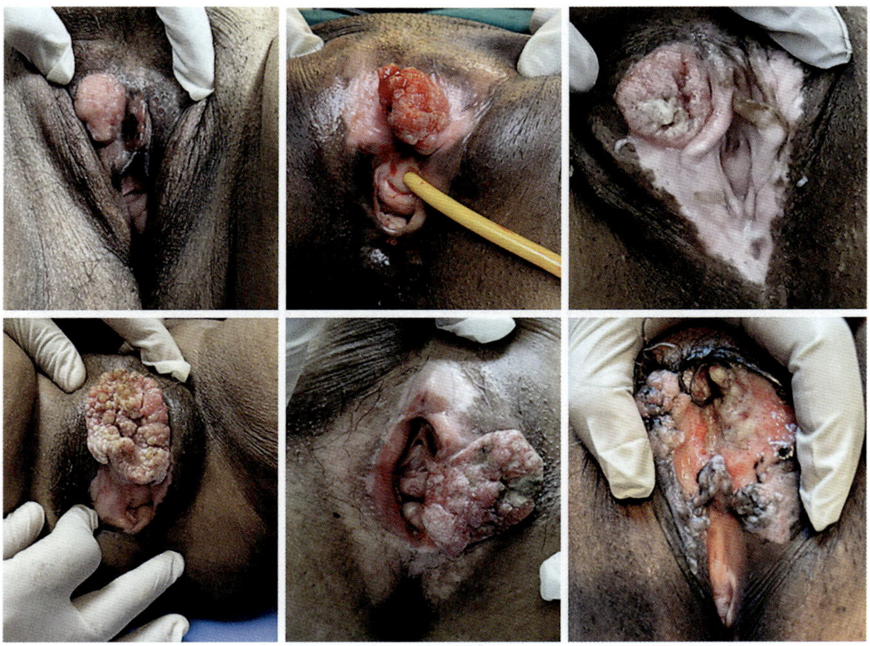

Fig. 1: Examples of vulvar carcinoma amenable to radical surgery.

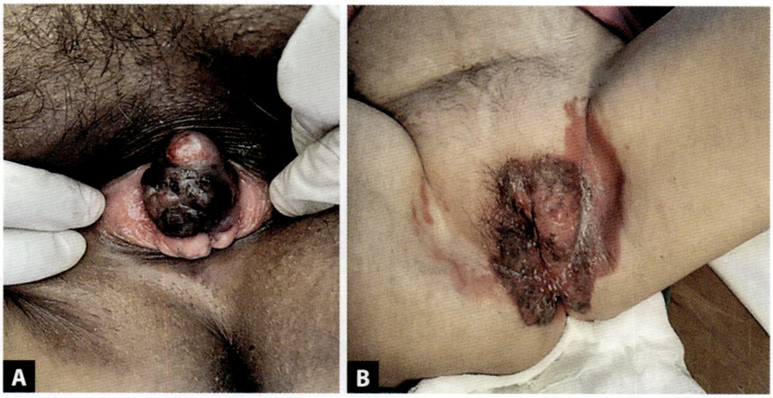

Figs. 2A and B: (A) Vulvar melanoma; (B) Paget's disease of vulva.

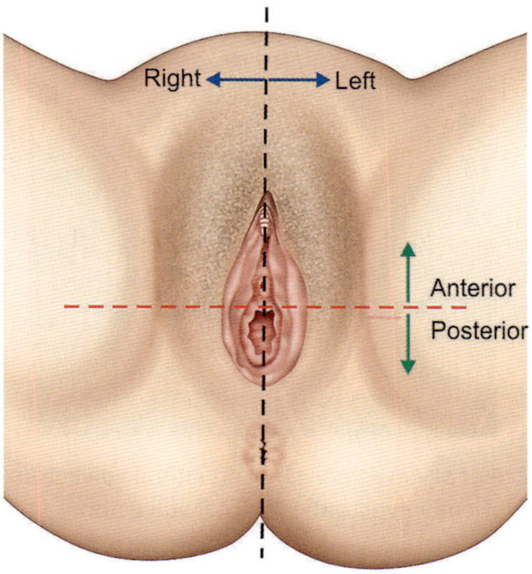

Fig. 3: Extent of vulvectomy.

TERMINOLOGIES

The International Society for the Study of Vulvovaginal Disease (ISSVD) in 2020 had proposed terminologies to bring about uniformity concerning surgeries for vulvar cancer.[1]

The extent of vulvectomy should be defined as **(Figs. 3 and 4)**:

- Total vulvectomy—when the entire vulva is excised.
- Partial vulvectomy—when only part of vulva is excised.
  - Lateral (right and left) excision—line connecting clitoris and anus divides vulva into right and left lateral areas.
  - Anterior and posterior excision—horizontal line drawn at the upper border of the hymenal ring divides vulva into anterior and posterior areas.

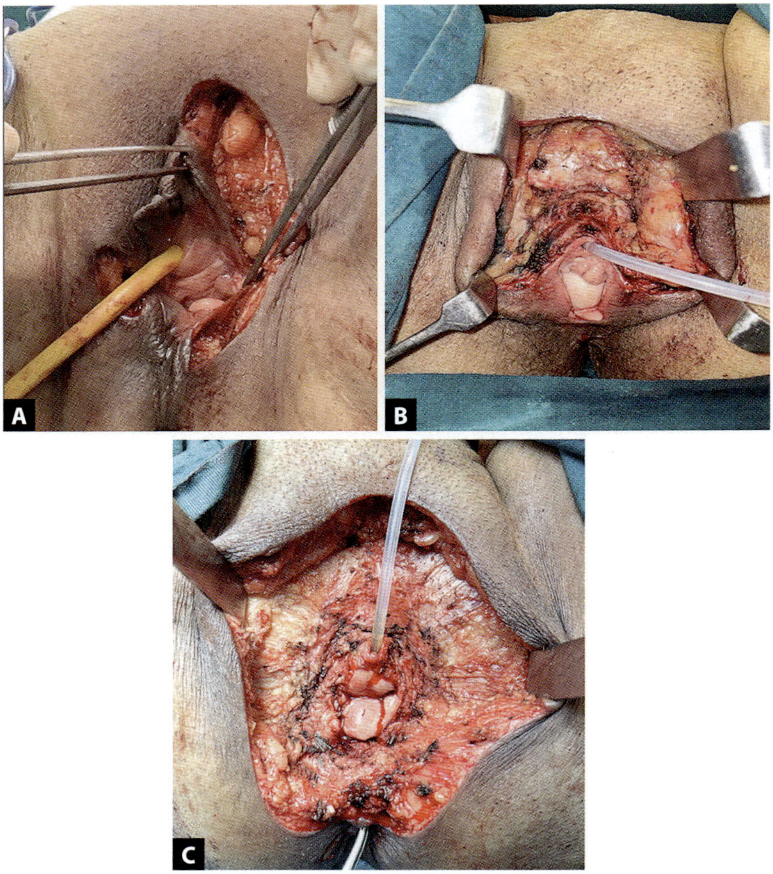

Figs. 4A to C: *Extent of vulvectomy:* (A) Left lateral vulvectomy; (B) Anterior hemivulvectomy; (C) Total vulvectomy.

The depth of vulvectomy is defined as:

- *Skinning or superficial:* Only skin/mucosa is excised leaving behind fatty tissue and fascial structures.
- *Simple:* Skin along with superficial portion of fatty tissue is excised.
- *Radical or deep*: Skin along with entire tissue beneath, extending up to the level of deep fascia of thigh, periosteum of pubic symphysis and inferior fascia of urogenital diaphragm is excised.

PREOPERATIVE EVALUATION

Vulval Biopsy

The indications for performing a vulval biopsy are:

- Any enlarging lesion or one that has changed color/appearance.
- Raised or pigmented lesion

- Vulvar dermatoses where the diagnosis is in doubt or there is no response to treatment.
- Any malignant appearing lesion
- Any lesion that has associated white or thickened areas.

The biopsy should be done from the edge of the lesion with a scalpel or Keyes punch biopsy forceps. The tissue should include underlying dermis and connective tissue so that the depth of stromal invasion can be evaluated.

INVESTIGATIONS

A thorough clinical examination (vulval mapping) must be done to assess local disease extent, involvement of urethra, vagina, anus and for any palpable inguinal nodes. Evaluation of cervix, vagina with pap smear and colposcopy should be done to rule out concomitant preinvasive/invasive lesions.

In case of suspicious involvement of urethra and anus, MRI pelvis, cystoscopy/proctoscopy should be done to know the extent of disease. For nodal status, USG of groins or CECT will be helpful. In case of suspicious nodes in clinical examination/preoperative imaging, FNAC/biopsy of the node will help to plan further management.

PREOPERATIVE COUNSELING AND SURGICAL CONSENT

Preoperative counseling and consenting are of utmost importance as vulvar surgeries may be associated with significant postoperative morbidity and may lead to gross distortion of perineal anatomy, resulting in ill perception of body image and effect on sexual function. While planning surgeries for lesions with proximity to urethra or anus, preoperative stoma (urostoma/colostoma) counseling is essential.

PROCEDURES

Radical Vulvectomy

- *Patient's position:* Patient is placed in lithotomy position with hip abducted 45° and flexed 45–90°. The perineum should be positioned to protrude over the end of the table. A Foley's catheter is placed.
- *Marking:* A marking ink is used to mark the planned incision. A 2 cm radial margin is marked with ruler from the gross margin of the tumor all around. The margin close to urethra and anus can be reduced to 1 cm **(Fig. 5)**.
- *Surgical procedure:* Skin and subcutaneous tissue are incised on the marked line and deepened to reach the inferior fascia of urogenital diaphragm. This should be done in a perpendicular fashion to avoid tunneling beneath the tumor, which will lead to shortening of the deep margin. Anterior traction is provided on the specimen and is detached from the fascia by using monopolar cautery.

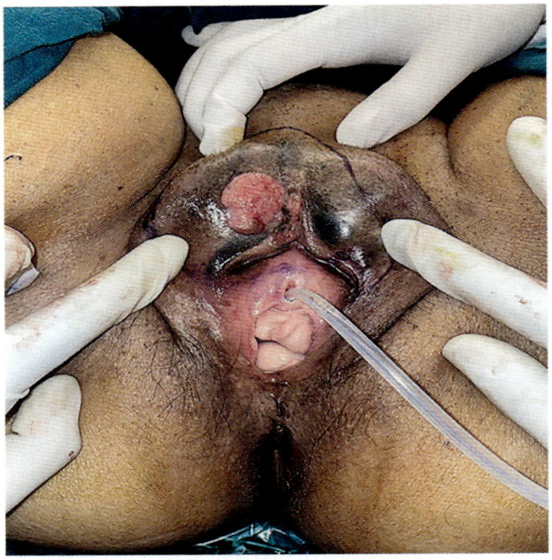

Fig. 5: Gross radial margin of 2 cm marked around the tumor.

During an interior dissection, the neurovascular bundle of the clitoris (in the suspensory ligament) may cause profuse bleeding. Therefore, it should be carefully isolated, clamped, transected, and ligated separately.

During posterior dissection, the vulval tissue is dissected from the perineal body and proceeded along the rectovaginal septum carefully. Anal sphincter injury can be prevented by placing a finger in the anus and guiding dissection accordingly. Branches of the internal pudendal artery are anticipated posterolaterally at 5 and 7 o'clock position.

Vaginal incision is made circumferentially on the marked line. Bleeding from venous sinuses around urethra and at vaginal introitus may be controlled by isolating the crura on both sides of clitoris, clamping, transecting and ligating them. Bulbocavernosus muscle and vestibular bulbs are also removed with the specimen. If tumor involves urethra, the distal 1–1.5 cm of the urethra can be removed without causing urinary incontinence **(Fig. 6)**.

Involvement of more than 1.5 cm of urethra, anterior and posterior vaginal wall or anal canal may require exenterative procedures **(Fig. 7)** and these patients are better treated with neoadjuvant chemotherapy/chemoradiotherapy or definitive chemoradiation followed by residual tumor excision.

DEFECT CLOSURE

- *Primary closure:* If the tissue surrounding the defect can be approximated without tension, then primary closure is preferred **(Fig. 8)**. After adequate hemostasis and copious irrigation, the subcutaneous tissue is closed with 3-0 delayed absorbable sutures. The vulvar margins are approximated with interrupted/continuous sutures (delayed absorbable/non-absorbable).

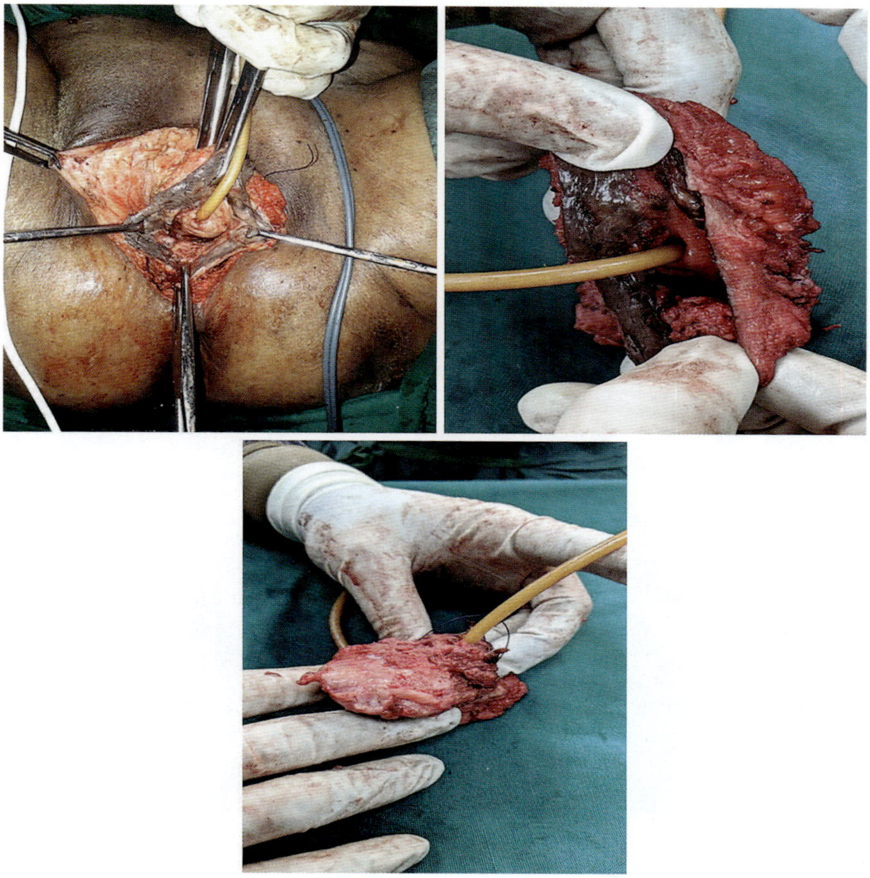

Fig. 6: Radical vulvectomy with distal urethrectomy.

Care is taken to avoid excess tension on the tissue. If the urethra has been resected, the cut end of urethral mucosa must be hitched to the surrounding tissue to prevent urethral retraction/misdirection/stenosis. It is preferable to avoid placing drain in the vulvar wound if the defect is not large.

- *Flap closure:* When defect is large and tissue mobilization is poor, then flaps may be required to close them. The type of flap employed depends on the site and extent of defect, vital structures resected and laxity of surrounding tissues[2] **(Table 1)**.

GROIN NODE DISSECTION

Indications

The indications and specifications of groin node dissection are summarized in **Table 2**.[3]

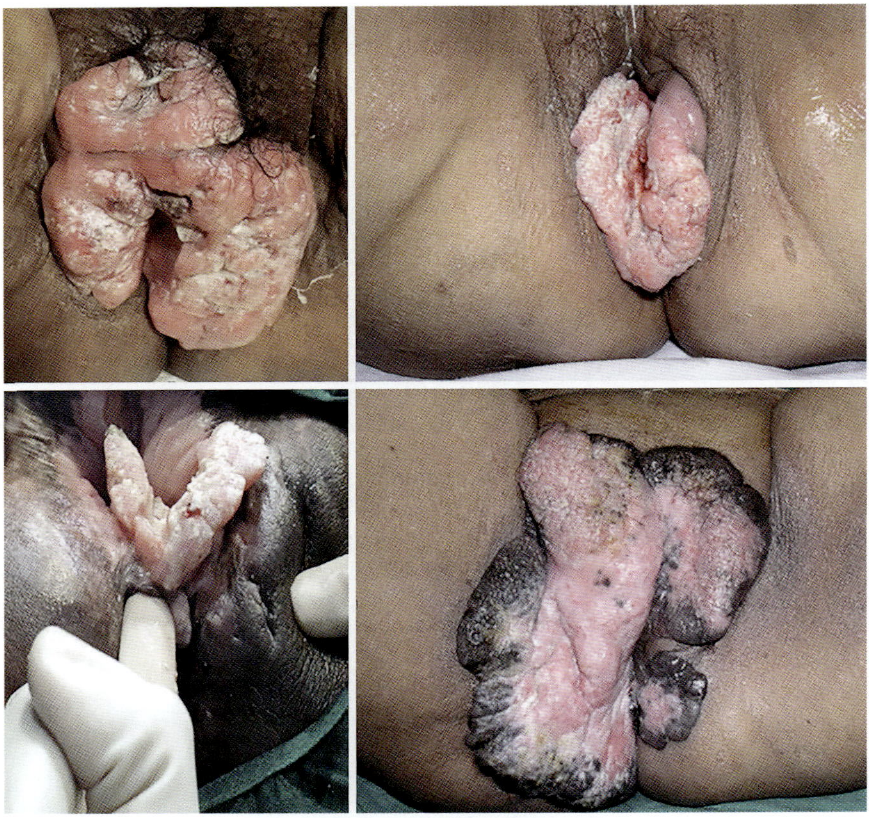

Fig. 7: Locally advanced cancers.

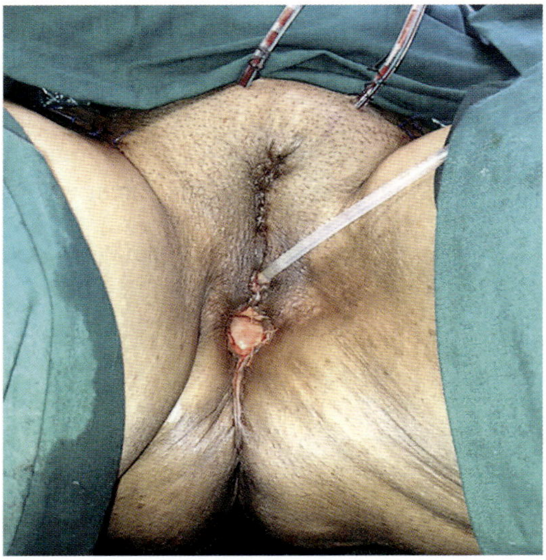

Fig. 8: Primary closure.

TABLE 1: Different types of flap closure.

Defect	*Flaps employed*	*Type of flap*
Vulvoperineal defect	• V to Y advancement flap **(Fig. 9)** • Lotus petal transposition flap **(Fig. 10)**	Fasciocutaneous
Vulvoperineal + groin defect	Anterolateral thigh flap **(Fig. 11)**	Fasciocutaneous or myocutaneous
Vulvoperineal + mons pubis defect	• Deep inferior epigastric perforator (DIEP) flap • Vertical rectus abdominis myocutaneous (VRAM) flap	Myocutaneous

TABLE 2: Indications for groin node dissection.

Primary lesion	*Groin node dissection (GND)*
Stage IA disease, i.e., T1 ≤2 cm with a depth of invasion ≤1.0 mm	No GND
Stage IB and II, lateral lesions	Ipsilateral GND
• Midline tumors • Involving anterior labia minora • Large lateral tumors • Positive nodes on ipsilateral side	Bilateral GND

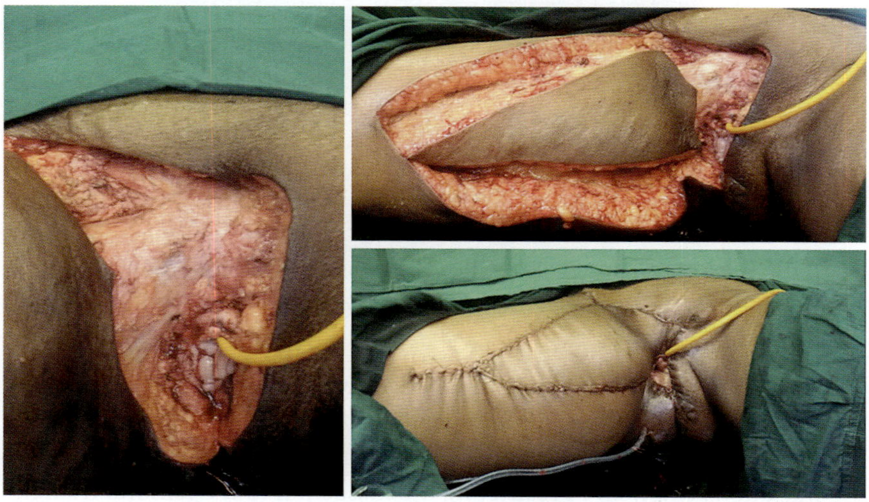

Fig. 9: V-Y advancement flap.

Procedure

Groin node dissection includes removal of superficial inguinal nodes above fascia lata and deep femoral nodes found beneath fascia lata along the femoral vessels. Removal of only superficial inguinal nodes has 6–8% local failure rate.[4] GND can be done prior to vulvectomy or simultaneously by two surgical teams.

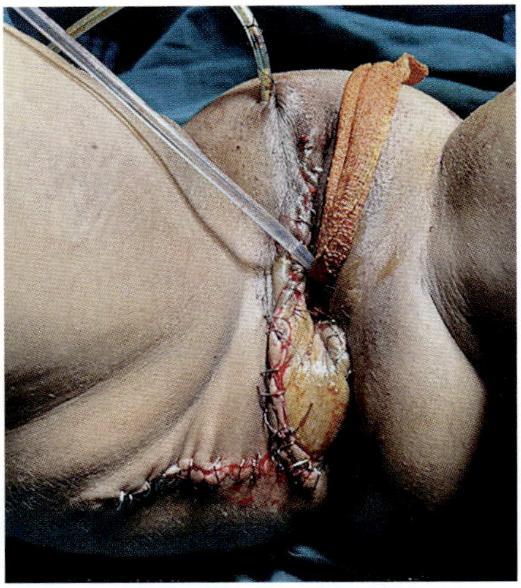

Fig. 10: Lotus petal transposition flap.

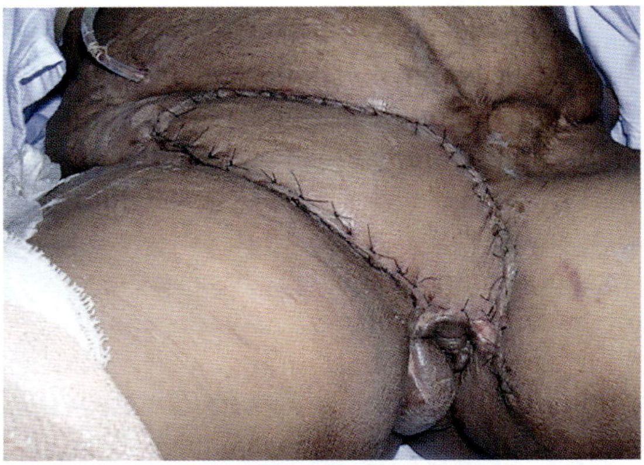

Fig. 11: Anterolateral thigh flap.

The skin incision is made in the medial two-thirds of a line drawn 2 cm below and parallel to the inguinal ligament extending from pubic tubercle to anterior superior iliac spine. Marking the course of femoral artery by feeling the pulsations can help in restricting the dissection to the femoral triangle. Care should be taken to make the incision away from the groin crease for better wound healing. The skin and subcutaneous layer are incised with a scalpel to expose the scarpa's fascia. Adequate thickness of the skin flaps should be maintained throughout to prevent flap necrosis. The scarpa's fascia is incised and an upward traction is applied to this fascia with Allis forceps or skin hooks.

Dissection is carried out below the scarpa's fascia cranially till the glistening silver-colored external oblique aponeurosis is reached. The

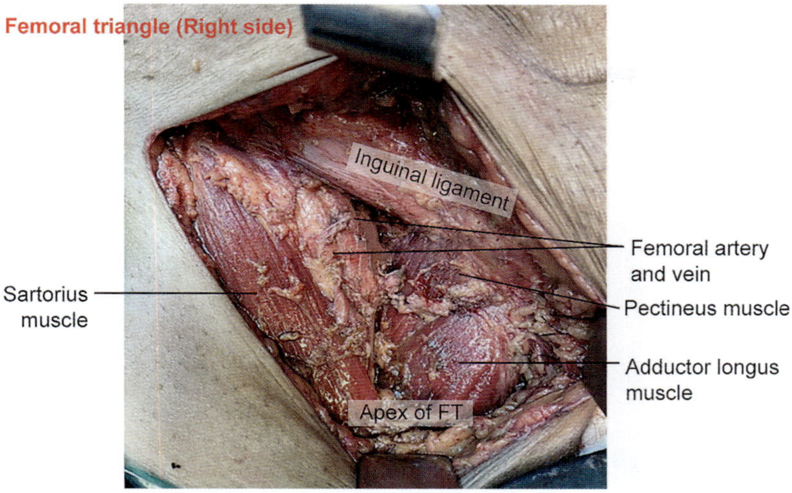

Fig. 12: Boundaries of groin node dissection.

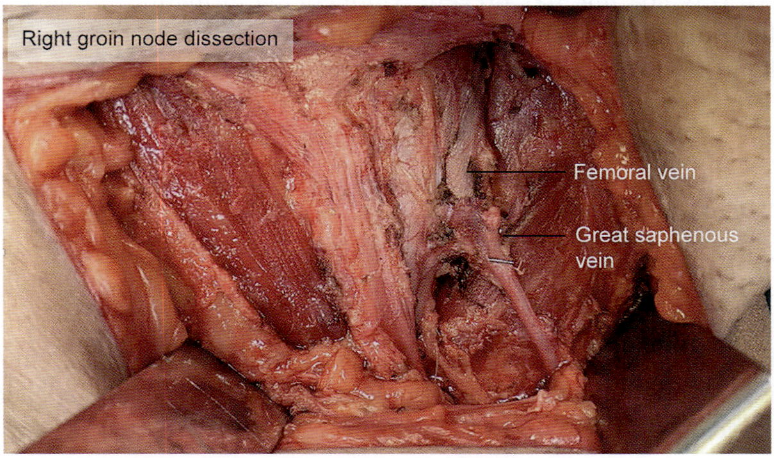

Fig. 13: Saphenous-sparing groin node dissection.

fatty tissue containing the superficial inguinal nodes is dissected off the inguinal ligament starting from lateral to medial direction. The dissection is carried out to expose cribriform fascia, fascia covering sartorius muscle laterally, fascia covering adductor longus muscle medially till the apex of femoral triangle **(Fig. 12)**. Superficial vessels—circumflex iliac, epigastric, external pudendal are encountered, that should be transected and ligated.

The great saphenous vein (GSV) is identified on the anteromedial side where it ascends and enters the saphenofemoral junction. The GSV is preserved usually (Saphenous-sparing GND) **(Fig. 13)**. Meta-analyses have

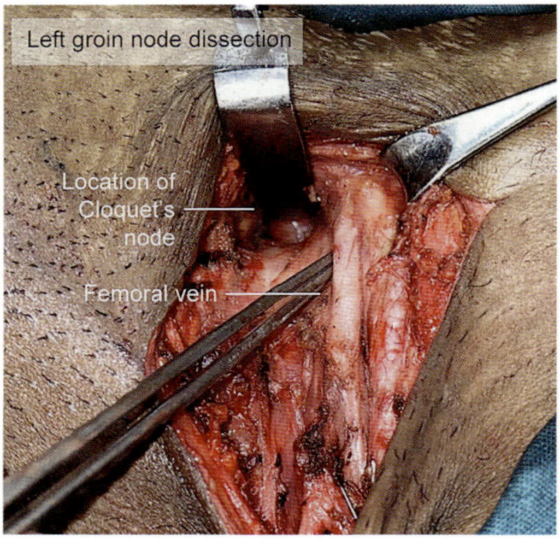

Fig. 14: Deep femoral node dissection.

shown GSV sparing may prevent lymphedema formation.[5] If needed to facilitate dissection, it can be ligated and transected at least 1 cm away from sapheno-femoral junction. Residual fibrofatty tissue anterior and medial to the femoral vein above the lower limit of fossa ovalis, that contains deep femoral node (Cloquet's node) is also removed **(Fig. 14)**.

Sartorius Transposition

A routine transposition of sartorius muscle is not recommended. However, if during dissection, excess deep fascia has been removed and the femoral vessels get exposed, or in cases with infected lymph nodes, a sartorius transposition can be done to cover femoral vessels. The sartorius muscle is divided from the anterior superior iliac spine using monopolar cautery, swung across the vessels and sutured to the inguinal ligament with absorbable sutures.

Closure of GND Wound

After a thorough wound wash, a closed suction drain is placed and brought out anterolaterally. The skin should be checked for viability, and it is preferable to refashion skin edges before closure. The scarpa's fascia is approximated with interrupted delayed absorbable sutures. The skin can be approximated with staplers or monofilament sutures **(Fig. 15)**. Care should be taken not place sutures too tightly that might lead to skin necrosis.

SENTINEL LYMPH NODE BIOPSY

Sentinel lymph node (SLN) brings down the rate of lymphedema from 64% to less than 2% when compared with complete inguinofemoral

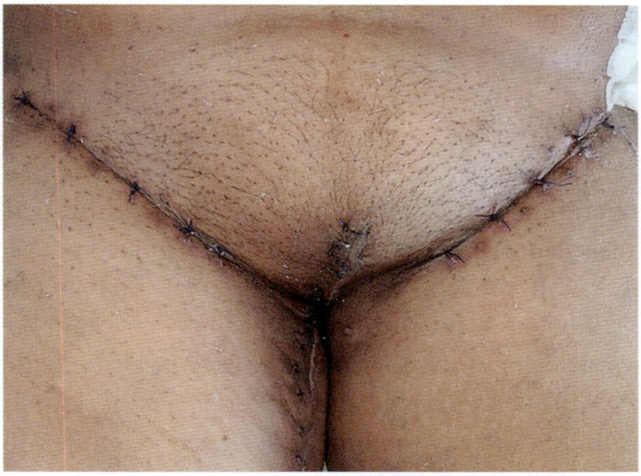

Fig. 15: Skin closure after groin node dissection.

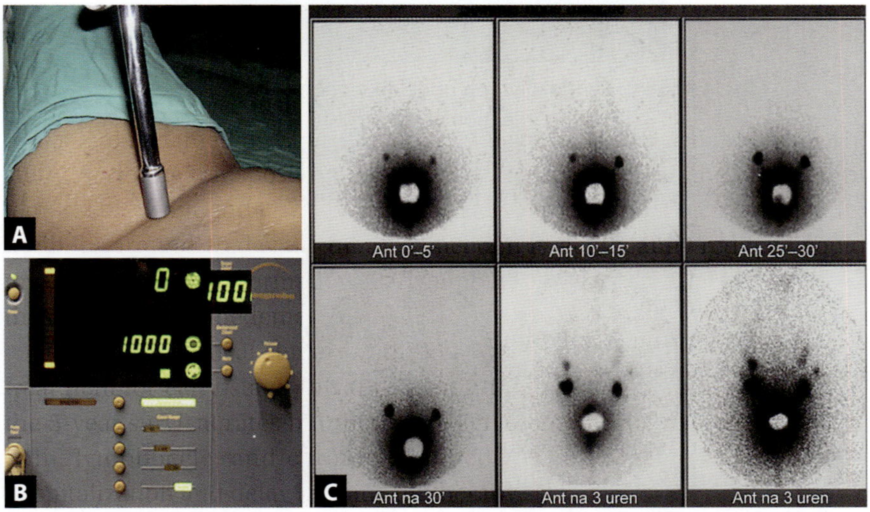

Figs. 16A to C: Radioactive tracer technique. Sentinel lymph node detection using Tc-99m. (A) Intraoperative use of gamma probe to localize sentinel node; (B) Gamma count display unit; (C) Preoperative lymphoscintigraphy.

lymphadenectomy.[6] SLND is recommended in unifocal, <4 cm tumors without suspicious nodes.[3]

The identification of sentinel lymph node is facilitated by:

- Preoperative (1 Day prior to 1–3 hours prior to surgery) four quadrant peritumoral intradermal injection of Tc-99m labeled colloids followed by lymphoscintigraphy which grossly localizes the sentinel node. Intraoperatively, gamma probe is used to identify the sentinel node and place incision accordingly **(Figs. 16A to C)**

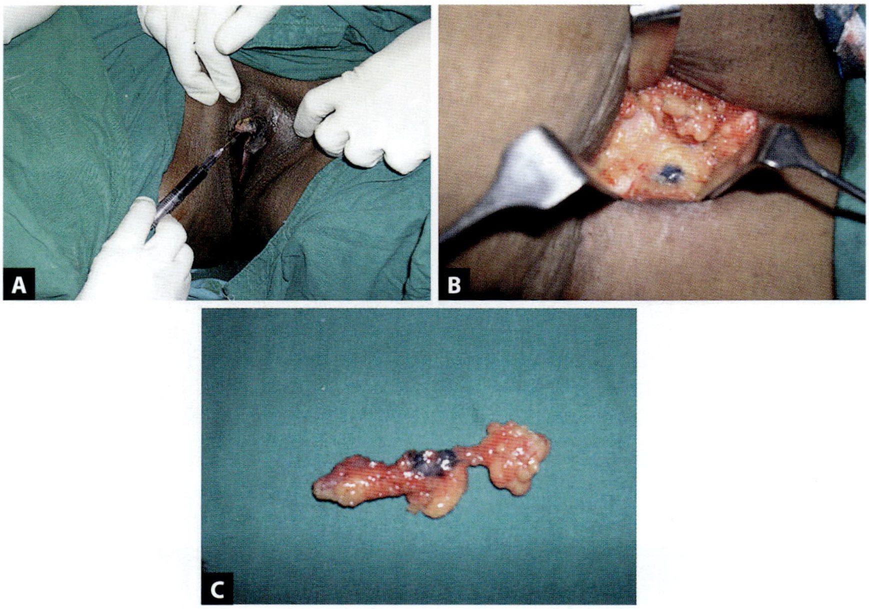

Figs. 17A to C: Sentinel lymph node dissection after intraoperative injection of blue dye.

- Intraoperative injection of isosulfan blue or methylene blue dye **(Figs. 17A to C)**
- Intraoperative injection of indocyanine green (ICG) dye and use of near infrared camera.

Dual technique (Tc-99m and blue dye/ICG) is recommended to improve detection rate. Any suspicious node apart from the sentinel node should also be removed. If no sentinel node is identified, then a complete inguinofemoral lymph node dissection must be done. In case of midline lesions, bilateral SLN detection is mandatory.

POSTOPERATIVE CARE

- Adequate intraoperative and postoperative antibiotic covers (including anaerobic cover) should be given because of high chances of wound contamination with stools.
- Thromboprophylaxis (mechanical and pharmacological) should be offered routinely.
- Good wound care—the wound should be always kept dry.
- Sitz bath can be started after few days of surgery to aid in vulvar wound healing.
- Laxatives can be added to avoid constipation.
- Groin drain removal is done once the output becomes less than 25 mL/24-hour.

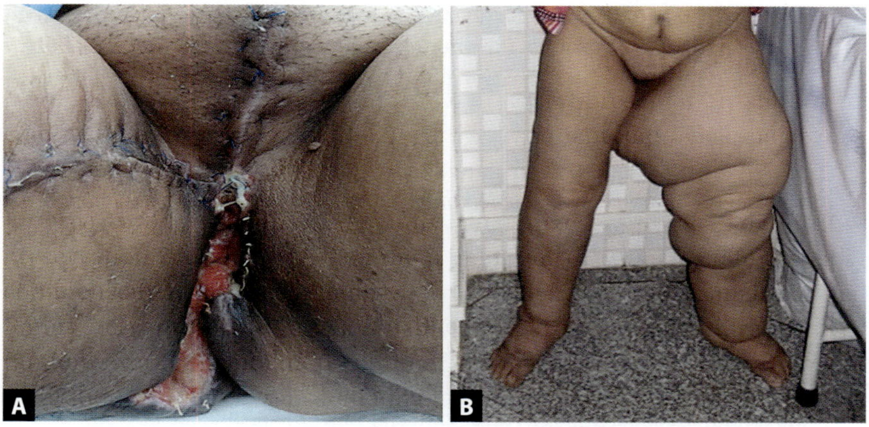

Figs. 18A and B: Postoperative complications. (A) Wound breakdown; (B) Lymphedema.

COMPLICATIONS

Intraoperative complications are relatively rare, but postoperative complication rates can be as high as 76% and are usually related to groin node dissection.[7]

- Lymphocyst formation (40%) is a common complication—mild in majority of patients and can be managed with tight compression dressings. Symptomatic lymphocysts need aspiration or may require placement of a drainage catheter.
- Infections (39%)—wound infections and UTI can occur frequently which are to be managed with antibiotics.
- Wound breakdown (17%) **(Fig. 18A)** is managed with daily dressing, appropriate antibiotics and sitz bath. Most wounds are left to heal by secondary intention.
- A significant long-term complication is lymphedema **(Fig. 18B)** and recurrent lymphangitis (28%). Apart from modifications in surgical techniques, postoperative use of compression stockings, limb elevation and exercises can be of help.

REFERENCES

1. Micheletti L, Haefner H, Zalewski K, MacLean A, Gomez Cherey F, Pereira C, Sluga C, Solé-Sedeno JM, Vargas-Hernandez VM, Preti M. The International Society for the Study of Vulvovaginal Disease Surgical Oncological Procedure Definitions Committee "Surgical Terminology for Vulvar Cancer Treatment". J Low Genit Tract Dis. 2020;24(1):62-8.
2. Gentileschi S, Servillo M, Garganese G, Fragomeni S, De Bonis F, Scambia G, Salgarello M. Surgical therapy of vulvar cancer: how to choose the correct reconstruction? J Gynecol Oncol. 2016;27(6):e60.

3. Oonk MHM, Planchamp F, Baldwin P, et al. European Society of Gynaecological Oncology Guidelines for the Management of Patients with Vulvar Cancer—Update 2023 International Journal of Gynecologic Cancer Published Online First: 27 June 2023.
4. Stehman FB, Bundy BN, Dvoretsky PM, Creasman WT. Early stage I carcinoma of the vulva treated with ipsilateral superficial inguinal lymphadenectomy and modified radical hemivulvectomy: a prospective study of the Gynecologic Oncology Group. Obstet Gynecol. 1992;79:490-7.
5. Tranoulis A, Laios A, Theophilou G, et al. The impact of saphenous vein sparing during inguinal lymphadenectomy on postoperative morbidity in women with vulval cancer: an updated per groin meta-analysis of short-term outcomes. International Journal of Gynecologic Cancer. 2018;28:1232-8.
6. Van der Zee AG, Oonk MH, De Hullu JA, et al. Sentinel node dissection is safe in the treatment of early-stage vulvar cancer. J Clin Oncol. 2008;26:884-9.
7. Gaarenstroom KN, Kenter GG, Trimbos JB, et al Postoperative complications after vulvectomy and inguinofemoral lymphadenectomy using separate groin incisions. International Journal of Gynecologic Cancer. 2003;13:522-7.

6

SECTION

Miscellaneous

17. **Breast Cancer Screening**
Karishma Kirti, Nita S Nair

18. **Colposcopy Manual**
Priya Ganesh Kumar, Kirti Shankhdhar

19. **Fertility Preservation in Gynecological Cancer**
Rohan Palshetkar, Nandita Palshetkar, Mayuri More, Chiranjeev Shetty

17

CHAPTER

Breast Cancer Screening

Karishma Kirti, Nita S Nair

The most common cancer in women worldwide is breast cancer. In India, 162,468 new cases of breast cancer were reported in the year 2018, making it the leading cause of cancer in women. 11.1% of cancer-related deaths were accounted by breast cancer in that year.[1] An urban rural divide in terms of breast cancer incidence has been noted and it is significant.[2] Screening helps identify unrecognized disease in an apparently healthy, asymptomatic individual. The method of screening may be done by tests, e.g., serum testing, imaging or examinations, whichever can be applied rapidly and easily for the target population. While screening may be limited by the accuracy of the method applied, overdiagnosis is also a problem as it leads to anxiety and strains the healthcare system. Mammography has become synonymous with breast cancer screening. But self-breast examination or clinical breast examination by a trained health professional can be considered, especially considering the available infrastructure.

The following are various screening modalities available for breast cancer screening:

- Breast self-examination (BSE)
- Clinical breast examination (CBE)
- Screening by imaging—mammogram/ultrasound/magnetic resonance imaging.

BREAST SELF-EXAMINATION

Breast self-examination is simple and does not involve expenses, hence it appears to be an ideal screening method. However, studies of its impact on mortality reduction are limited. Shanghai trial[3] and Russian trial[4] were two landmark randomized trial that tried to assess the efficacy of BSE as screening method. The Shanghai trial recruited 266,064 factory workers and study population were randomly assigned to BSE instruction and non-instruction group. No significant differences were noted in the two groups in terms of tumor size, stage and cumulative breast cancer mortality rates.

There was no reduction in breast cancer mortality rates but there was a definite increase in detection of smaller benign breast lumps. The Russia trial did not fare much differently in terms of impact on mortality reduction. The study population were 122,471 women, who were assigned randomly to BSE or no BSE groups. A positive impact noted was slightly higher survival rate in the BSE group (53.2% vs. 45.8%, $p = 0.051$). In the experimental arm, the indications for biopsy were more than double (7.5% vs. 3.5%, $p < 0.01$). These findings were mirrored in a meta-analysis done by Hackshaw, et al.[5] The analysis concluded that there was no impact on the breast cancer mortality and noted that compliance was low and participation in the BSE teaching classes were low. The upside of these studies was then there was increased awareness about breast cancer and overall breast health.

CLINICAL BREAST EXAMINATION

Clinical breast examination involves examination by a well-trained healthcare professional. Mammography has been used as an effective screening tool, but over the years, it has faced criticisms as in premenopausal women, it has shown low sensitivity. Mammography alone or in combination with CBE when used for screening in women 50 years and above, resulted in reduction cause-specific mortality. The problem, however, was that this resulted in approximately 25% overdiagnosis after 25 years of follow-up.[6] Pisani, et al.[7], Sankarnarayanan, et al.[8] and Mittra, et al.[9] conducted randomized controlled trials evaluating the role of CBE in screening for breast cancer. Pisani, et al. used trained nurses/midwives to conduct the CBE. 151,168 women aged 35–64 years, also trained in SBE, were recruited, and assigned randomly to CBE versus no CBE groups. Compliance was poor despite home visits for those who were screened positive, and the study was discontinued after the first round of screening. Sankarnarayanan, et al. recruited 115,652 healthy women aged 30–69 years and randomized them to CBE and no screening groups. The percentage of early-stage (stage IIA or lower) breast cancers detected in the intervention was 43.8% vs. control groups 25.4% (P = 0.023). Advanced-stage (stage IIB or higher) disease detected were 45.0% in the intervention group vs. 68.3% (P = 0.005) in the no intervention group; thus, a downstaging of cancers was noted in the CBE arm. Mitra, et al. conducted a 20 years' prospective cluster-randomized trial, recruiting 151,538 women aged 36–64 years with no prior history of breast cancer. The intervention group had significant downstaging at diagnosis. There was a notable 30% reduction in mortality, but it was not significant **(Table 1)**.

IMAGING MODALITIES

Aside from mammography (MMG), ultrasound (US), and magnetic resonance imaging (MRI) are used for screening of breast cancer. Incorporation of

TABLE 1: Efficacy of randomized controlled studies for combined modality breast cancer screening (MMG and CBE).

Study	*Cancers detected in the screened population*	*Interval cancers*	*CBE*		*Downstaging*	
			Sensitivity	*Specificity*	*Screened*	*Control*
Mumbai study	73	37	57.44%	91.99%	• Early 78 • Advanced 38	• Early 32 • Advanced 37
Philippines study	68	NA	53.2%	100%	17% more advanced cases in control group	
Trivandrum study	80	28	54.1%	94%	• Early 43.8 • Advanced 45.0	• Early 25.4 • Advanced 68.3

artificial intelligence into screening mammography is being explored nowadays. Efficacy of mammography for breast cancer detection has been investigated in numerous randomized controlled trials (RCTs). The Health Insurance Plan (HIP) study[10] recruited 6200 women aged 40–64 years and used MMG and CBE by trained surgeons for screening. Follow-up after 18 years showed a relative risk (RR) of 0.77 (0.52–1.13) for women aged 40–49 for breast cancer mortality and 0.79 (0.58–1.08) for women aged 50–64, with an overall RR of 0.78 (0.61–1.00). Various screening trials have been done since then—the Edinburgh Randomized Trial[11] of Breast Cancer Screening; Canadian National Breast Screening Study I and II;[12,13] UK Age trial,[14] The Malmö Trial,[15] Swedish Two-County Trial;[16] and Göteborg Breast Screening Trial[17] **(Table 2)**. The variations in the findings of these studies were reviewed by Olsen and Gotzsche.[18,19] It was a landmark review, categorizing the studies into adequately and suboptimally randomized studies **(Table 3)**. There was no reduction in breast cancer mortality at 7 or 13 years (RR 0.90, CI 0.79–1.02), if the adequately randomized studies only were considered. But when the inadequately randomized trials were incorporated into the analysis, both 7 and 13-year reductions in breast cancer mortality significantly decreased (RR 0.75). With overall RR for all 7 trials at 0.81, the review emphasized on breast cancer mortality as an unreliable outcome and was in favor of screening. In conclusion, they highlighted that for every 2000 women invited for screening throughout 10 years, one would avoid dying from breast cancer, while 10 healthy women, who would have remained undiagnosed without screening, would undergo unnecessary treatment.

TABLE 2: Screening details of the randomized trials of breast cancer screening using mammography.

Study	*Year*	*Age at entry*	*Numbers screened*		*Screening Interval and rounds of screening 5 rounds*	*Available follow-up*
			Screened	*Control*	*MMG + CBE vs CBE/not and no of rounds of screening*	
HIP	1963–1969	40–64	31000	31000	Annual MMG + CBE vs not 3 rounds	18 years
Edinburgh	1978–1991	45–64	22944	21344	2 yearly MMG + annual CBE (7 rounds)	10 years
CNBSS I	1980	40–49	44925	44910	Annual MMG + CBE + BSE Vs One time CBE + BSE at initial evaluation	25 years
CNBSS II	1980	50–59			Annual MMG + CBE + BSE Vs Annual CBE + BSE	25 years
UK Age trial	1990–1997	39–41	53883	106953	Annual MMG	22·8 years
Malmö I	1976–1978	45–70 years	21088	21195	MMG every 18–24 months (5 rounds)	30 years
Malmö II	1978–1990	43–49	9587	8199	MMG every 18–24 months	22 years
Swedish two county trial	1977–1979	40–74	77080	55985	• 40–49 years—MMG every 2 years • 50–74 years—MMG every 3 years	29 years
Stockholm trial	1981–1985	40–64 years	40318	20000	MMG every 2 years (2 rounds)	25 years
Göteborg trial	1982–1991	39–59	21650	29961	MMG every 18 months (5 rounds)	25 years

TABLE 3: Cochrane Review 2021, a landmark review carried out by Olsen and Gøtzsche.

Adequately randomized	*Suboptimally randomized*
Malmö I trial	New York HIP trial
Canadian trial	Malmö II trial
UK age trial	Swedish 2 county trial
	Göteborg trial
	Stockholm trial
	Edinburgh trial—not included

TABLE 4: ACR-BI RADS categories.

5th edition		*Likelihood of cancer*
Category 0	Incomplete—additional imaging needed	N/A
Category 1	Negative	Essentially 0%
Category 2	Benign	Essentially 0%
Category 3	Probably benign	0 to ≤2%
Category 4	Suspicious	
4a	Low suspicion of malignancy	>2 to ≤10%
4b	Moderate suspicion of malignancy	>10 to ≤50%
4c	High suspicion of malignancy	>50 to <95%
Category 5	Highly suggestive of malignancy	≥95%
Category 6	Known biopsy-proven malignancy	N/A

Ultrasound

Ultrasound is also one of the modalities used for breast cancer screening. The combination of mammography and ultrasound for screening of breast cancer has shown increased sensitivity, high false positives and increased biopsy rates are unacceptable. In women with elevated risk of breast cancer, the addition of a single screening ultrasound to mammography will yield an additional 1.1–7.2 cancers per 1000 high-risk women; however, it also substantially increases the number of false positives.[20] USG can at best serve as an additional tool to mammography screening in women with intermediate risk for breast cancer (personal history of breast cancer or biopsies associated with increased risk or relative with early onset breast cancer).[21] USG-detected lesions is interpreted by categorizing the lesions into BI-RADS scoring **(Table 4)**.

For patients at higher-than-average risk for breast cancer, MRI has proven to be more sensitive than MMG. MRI for screening of breast cancer is universally recommended for women who are BRCA1/BRCA2 positive and for those with a higher than 25% lifetime risk of breast cancer. MRI as supplemental screening in women at an average risk of breast cancer (lifetime risk <15%) was assessed in a German study and found that MRI helped identify additional breast cancers that were not detected with MMG or USG, with an additional cancer yield of 15.5 per 1000 cases. These additional cancers diagnosed were small in size (median 8 mm), mostly node negative (93%) and tended to exhibit an adverse biological profile. The rate of interval cancer was zero. The study group suggested the use of MRI as a supplemental tool for average-risk women, especially those with dense breasts.

Artificial intelligence (AI) incorporation into screening mammography shows great potential for improving breast cancer detection, minimizing false positives, and streamlining the efficiency of breast cancer screening programs. Compared to traditional radiologist interpretation, the clinical safety of AI-supported mammography screening was evaluated in a randomized trial conducted in Sweden.[22] 80,033 women were recruited; the AI-supported screening detected 244 cases of cancer which implied detection of 6.1 per 1000 participants, thus, meeting safety benchmarks. On the other hand, the standard screening identification rate was 5.1 per 1000. Recall rates, false positive rates, and positive predictive values remained similar between the two methods. AI has significantly reduced the workload associated with screening by 44.3%. This study demonstrated the safety and efficacy of AI integration in mammography screening, maintaining a comparable cancer detection rate while enhancing efficiency. The trial continues to monitor interval cancer rates in a cohort of 100,000 participants during a 2-year follow-up period.

The efficacy of screening can be evaluated in terms of downstaging, chances of overdiagnosis, adverse effects and cost effectiveness. Detection of disease in early-stage facilitates timely intervention and treatment. Screening studies have shown increased incidence in intervention arm compared to control arm. Although the lesions in screened arm were early staged disease, no difference in mortality noted. If the intervention can definitively demonstrate the downstaging of breast cancer, impact on breast cancer-related mortality can be expected. With mammography, overdiagnosis is a significant drawback and supplementing with CBE may help reduce it. Adverse effects of screening are related to false diagnosis. Women may have psychological anxiety and testing itself carries certain morbidity. Cost and cost effectiveness of screening strategies were evaluated by Sarvazyan, et al. in addition to the diagnostic accuracy. The study group concluded that clinical breast examination has the potential for providing effective screening for breast cancer, especially considering countries with limited resources.[23]

Hence, BSE is useful as an awareness tool, CBE is effective for down-staging and imaging modalities as screening method have reduced mortality in women over 50 years of age.

REFERENCES

1. Bray F, et al. Global Cancer Statistics 2018: GLOBOCAN estimates of incidence and mortality worldwide for 36 cancers in 185 countries. CA Cancer J Clin. 2018;68(6):394-424.
2. Nagrani RT, Budukh A, Koyande S, Panse NS, Mhatre SS, Badwe R. Rural urban differences in breast cancer in India. Indian J Cancer. 2014;51:277-81.
3. Thomas DB, Gao DL, Ray RM, et al. Randomized trial of breast self-examination in Shanghai: final results. J Nat Cancer Inst. 2002;94: 1445-57.
4. Semiglazov VF, Manikhas AG, Moiseenko VM, et al. Results of a prospective randomised investigation [Russia (St Petersburg)/WHO] to evaluate the significance of self-examination for the early detection of breast cancer. Vopr Onkol. 2003;49:434-41.
5. Hackshaw A, Paul E. Breast self-examination and death from breast cancer: a meta-analysis. Br J Cancer. 2003;88:1047-95. doi: 10.1038/sj.bjc.6600847.
6. Kalager M, Adami HO, Bretthauer M, Tamimi RM. Overdiagnosis of invasive breast cancer due to mammography screening: results from the Norwegian screening program. Ann Intern Med. 2012; 156:491-9. doi: 10.7326/0003-4819-156-7-201204030-00005.
7. Pisani P, Parkin DM, Ngelangel C, et al. Outcome of screening by clinical examination of the breast in a trial in the Philippines. Int J Cancer. 2006;118(1): 149-54.
8. Sankarnarayanan R, Ramdas K, Thara S, et al. Clinical breast examination: preliminary results form a cluster randomised controlled trial in India. J Natl cancer Inst. 2011;103(19):1476-80.
9. Mittra I, Mishra GA, Dikshit RP, et al. Effect of screening by clinical breast examination on breast cancer incidence and mortality after 20 years: prospective, cluster randomised controlled trial in Mumbai. [published correction appears in BMJ. 2021 Mar 19;372:n738]. BMJ. 2021;372:n256. Published 2021 Feb 24. doi:10.1136/bmj.n256.
10. Shapiro S, Strax P, Venet L. Periodic breast cancer screening in reducing mortality from breast cancer. JAMA. 1971;215:1777-85.
11. Alexander FE. The Edinburgh Randomised Trial of Breast Cancer Screening. J Natl Cancer Inst Monogr. 1997;22:31-5.
12. Miller AB, Baines CJ, To T, Wall, C. Canadian National Breast Screening Study: 2. Breast cancer detection in death rates among women aged 50 to 59 years. CMAJ. 1992;147:1477-88.
13. Miller AB, et al. Twenty-five year follow up for breast cancer incidence and mortality of the Canadian Nation Breast Cancer Screening Study: randomised screening trial. BMJ. 2014;348:g366.
14. Moss SM, et al. Effect of mammographic screening from age 40 years on breast cancer mortality in the UK Age Trial at 17 years' follow-up: a randomised controlled trial. Lancet Oncol. 2015;16: 1123-32.
15. Andersson I, Aspegren K, Janzon L, et al. Mammographic screening and mortality from breast cancer: the Malmö mammographic screening trial. BMJ. 1988;297:943-8.

16. Tabar L, Vitak B, Chen TH, et al. Swedish two-county trial: Impact of mammographic screening on breast cancer mortality during 3 decades. Radiol. 2011;260(3):658-63.
17. Bjurstam N, Björneld L, Duffy SW, et al. The Gothenburg breast screening trial. Cancer. 1997;80:2091-9.
18. Olsen O, Gøtzsche PC. Cochrane review on screening for breast cancer with mammography. Lancet. 2001;358:1340-2.
19. Gøtzsche PC, Jørgensen KL. Screening for breast cancer with mammography. Cochrane Library. https://doi.org/10.1002/14651858.CD001877.pub5.
20. Berg WA, Blume JD, Cormack JB, et al. Combined screening with ultrasound and mammography vs mammography alone in women at elevated risk of breast cancer. JAMA. 2008;299(18):2151-63.
21. Kuhl CK, Strobel K, Bieling H, et al. Supplemental breast MR imaging screening of women with average risk of breast cancer. Radiol. 2017;283(2):361-70.
22. Lång K, Josefsson V, Larsson AM, et al. Artificial intelligence-supported screen reading versus standard double reading in the Mammography Screening with Artificial Intelligence trial (MASAI): a clinical safety analysis of a randomised, controlled, non-inferiority, single-blinded, screening accuracy study. Lancet Oncol. 2023;24(8):936-44. doi:10.1016/S1470-2045(23)00298-X.
23. Sarvazyan A, Egorov V, Son JS, Kaufman CS. Cost-effective Screening for Breast Cancer Worldwide: Current State and Future Directions. Breast Cancer (Auckl). 2008;1:91-9.

18 CHAPTER

Colposcopy Manual

Priya Ganesh Kumar, Kirti Shankhdhar

Colposcopy is the examination of cervix, vagina and vulva under adequate illumination and magnification **(Fig. 1)**. The magnification used is between 5 and 20 x.

PURPOSE

- Detect intraepithelial neoplasia of cervix
- Diagnose lesions due to human papillomavirus (HPV) infection
- Detect early neoplasia of cervix, vagina, and vulva

INDICATIONS OF COLPOSCOPY

- Abnormal screening test
- Positive HR-HPV test
- *Cytological abnormalities*: LSIL, ASCUS (HPV +ve or X2), ACS-H, HSIL, AGC/AIS, carcinoma

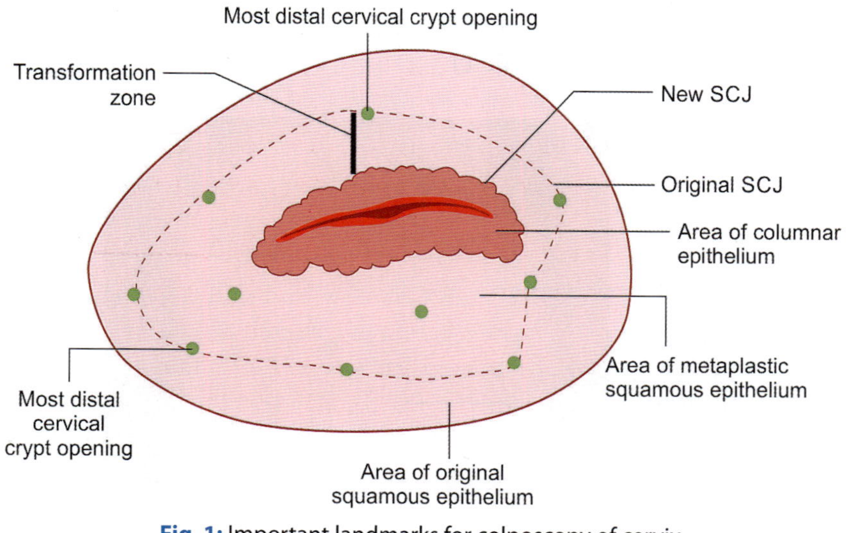

Fig. 1: Important landmarks for colposcopy of cervix.

- Positive VIA test
- Abnormal cervix
- Postcoital bleeding
- Post-treatment follow-up
- Vulval, vaginal lesions

TISSUE BASIS OF COLPOSCOPY OF CERVIX

- Colposcopy is based on variable absorption and reflection of white light off different tissue interfaces.
- Colposcope allows magnification and illumination of cervix.
- By applying 5% acetic acid and Lugol's iodine to the cervix, abnormalities can be identified including benign, precancerous, and malignant changes **(Fig. 2)**.

PROCEDURE OF COLPOSCOPY

- Counseling
- Consent
- Pass the Cusco speculum under supervision **(Fig. 3)**
- Take the samples (Pap/HPV DNA/LBC) **(Fig. 4)**
- *Access adequacy:*
  - TZ type (TZ or transformation zone is area between original squamocolumnar junction and new squamocolumnar junction) **(Figs. 5 to 7)**.
  - Application of 3–5% acetic acid for one minute (Due to higher protein content in nucleus precancerous and cancerous cells turn acetowhite) helps to:
  - Determine TZ **(Fig. 8)**
  - Application of Lugol's iodine **(Fig. 9)**
- Calculate Swede Score **(Table 1)**

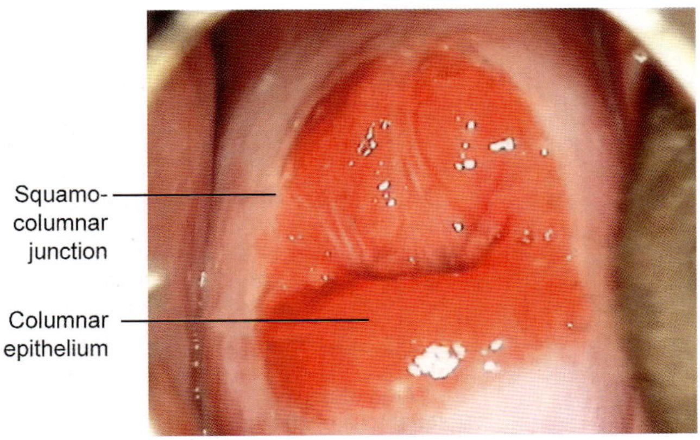

Fig. 2: Colposcopy of cervix.

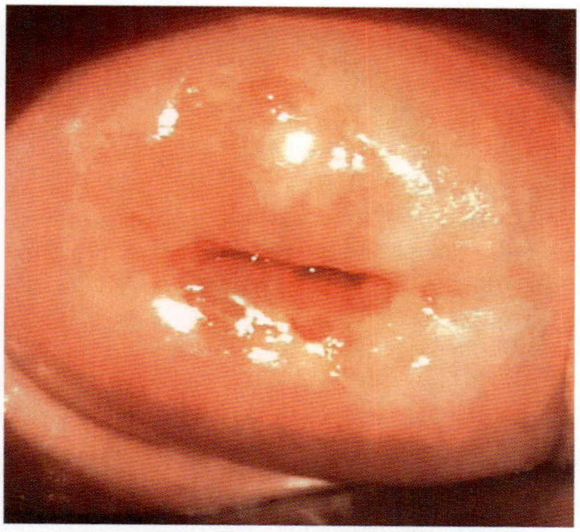

Fig. 3: The cervix is exposed used a bivalve speculum without use of lubricant.

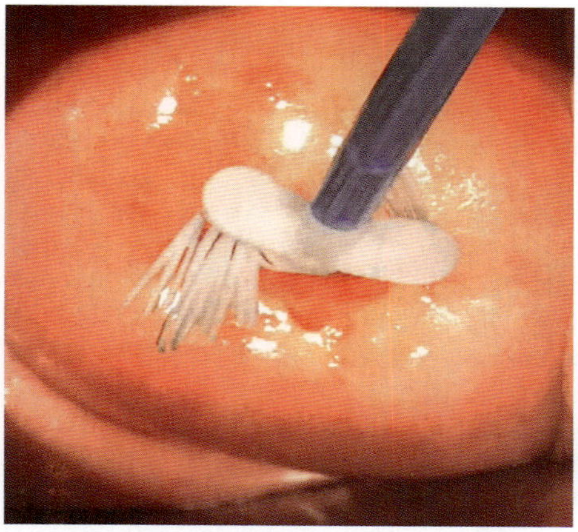

Fig. 4: The brush is inserted into the endocervical canal as shown and rotated clockwise three times. Alternatively, Ayre spatula and endocervical brush can be used for collection of Pap smear.

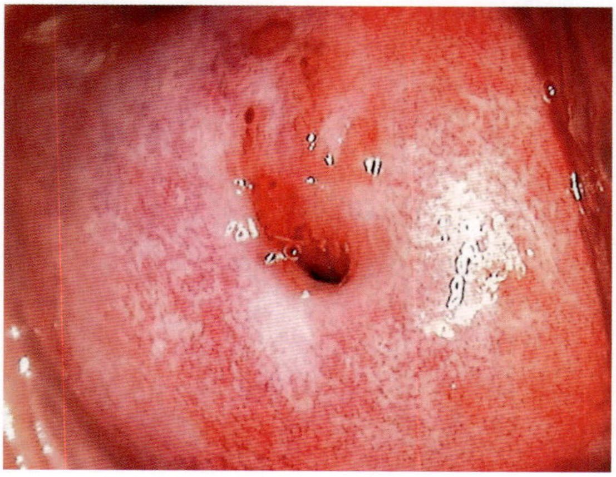

Fig. 5: TZ1–SCJ completely visual.

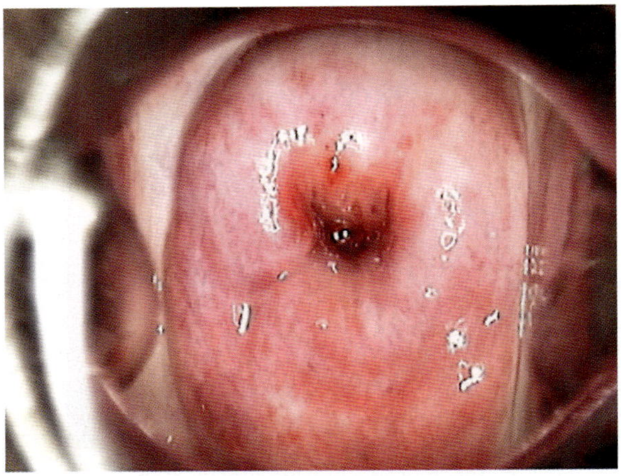

Fig. 6: TZ2–SCJ partially visual.

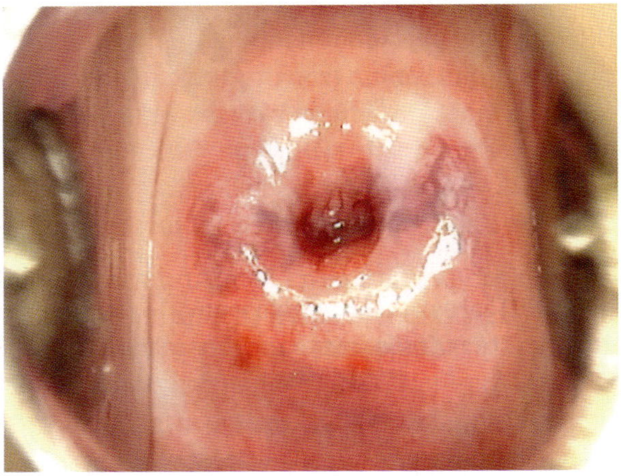

Fig. 7: TZ3–SCJ not visual.

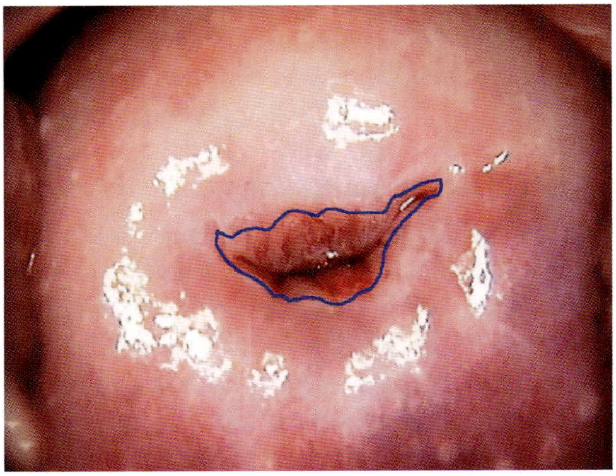

Fig. 8: Identifying TZ.

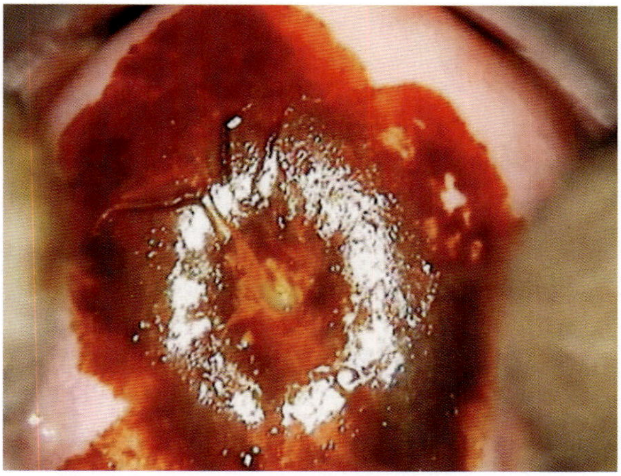

Fig. 9: Due to higher glycogen in cytoplasm of cells, mature squamous epithelium turn dark brown.

TABLE 1: Swede score.

Characteristics	*0*	*1*	*2*
Aceto uptake	Zero or transparent	Shady, milky (not transparent, not opaque)	Distinct, opaque white
Margins/ surfaces	Diffuse	Sharp but irregular, jagged, geographical satellites	Sharp and even, difference in surface level including cuffing
Vessels	Fine, regular	Absent	Coarse or typical
Lesion size	<5 mm	5–15 mm or spanning two quadrants	>15 or 3–4 quadrants or endocervically undefined
Iodine staining	Brown	Faintly or patchy yellow	Distinct yellow

ABNORMAL COLPOSCOPIC FINDING

- Ectopy **(Figs. 10 to 12)**
- Metaplasia **(Figs. 13 to 15)**
- Low-grade lesions **(Figs. 16 to 18)**
- High-grade lesions **(Figs. 19 to 21)**

TREATMENT

Principles of treatment:

- Entire CIN lesion should be treated.
- The minimum depth of treatment should be 7 mm.
- Proper follow-up of all treated patients to diagnose recurrence.

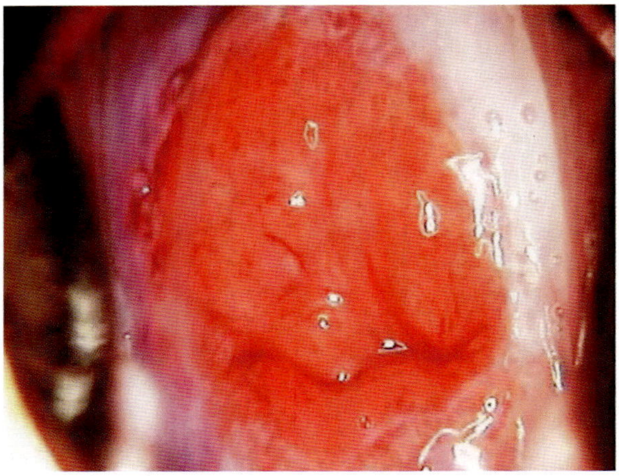

Fig. 10: After normal saline for ectopy.

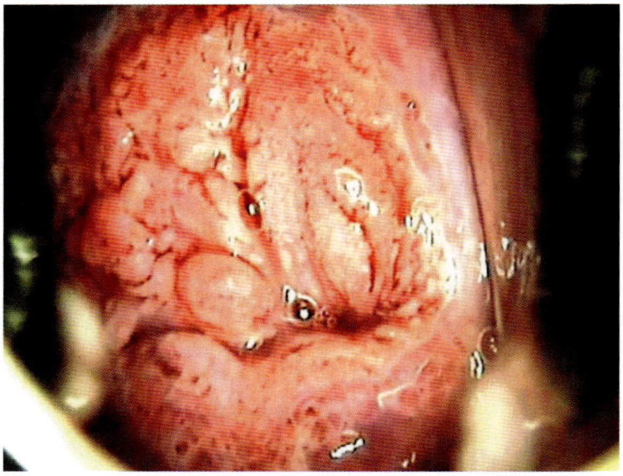

Fig. 11: After acidic acid for ectopy.

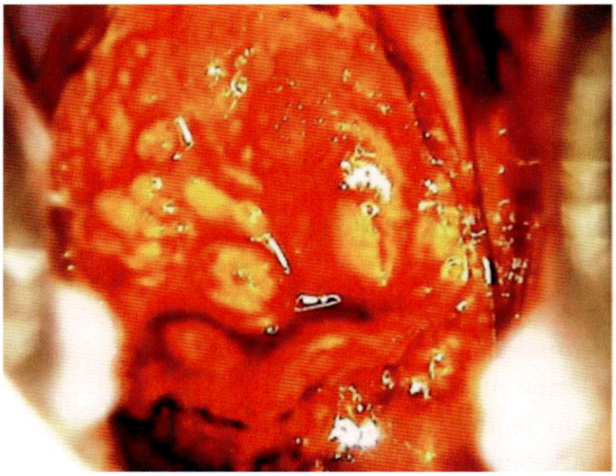

Fig. 12: After Lugol's iodine for ectopy.

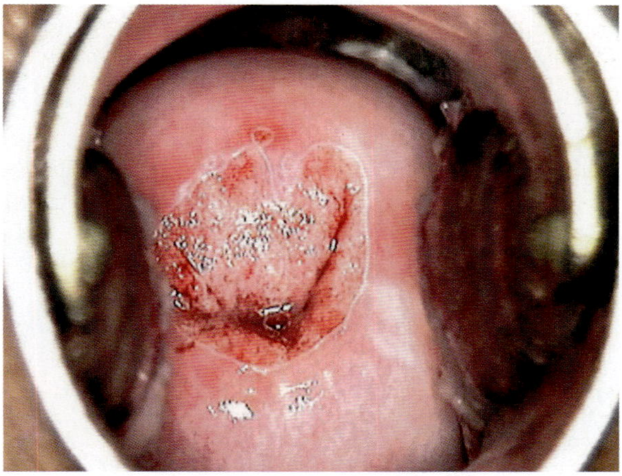

Fig. 13: After normal saline for metaplasia.

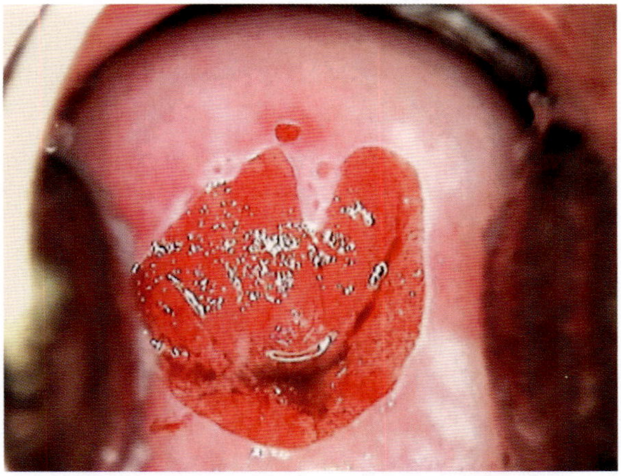

Fig. 14: After acidic acid for metaplasia.

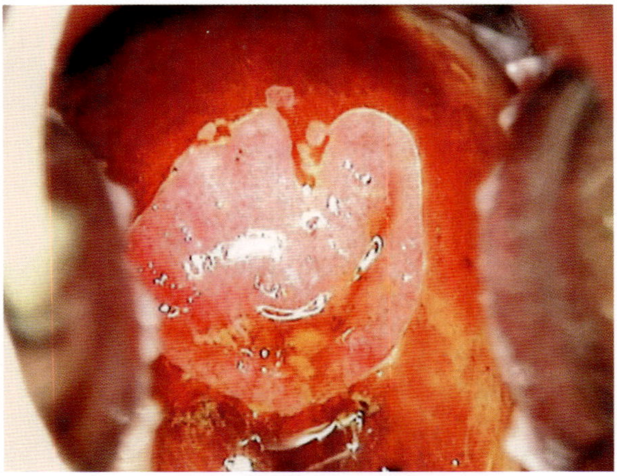

Fig. 15: After Lugol's iodine for metaplasia.

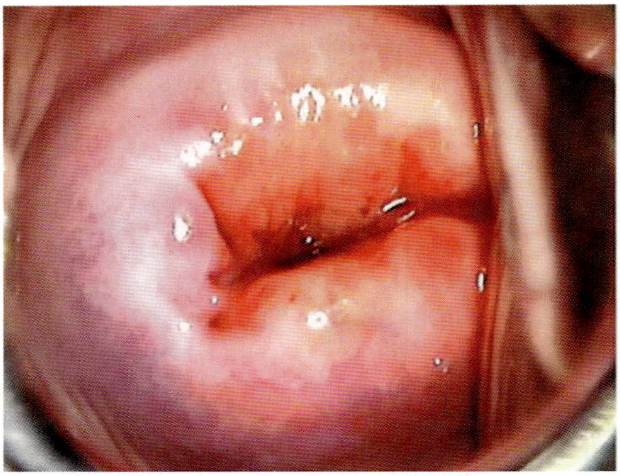

Fig. 16: After normal saline for low-grade lesions.

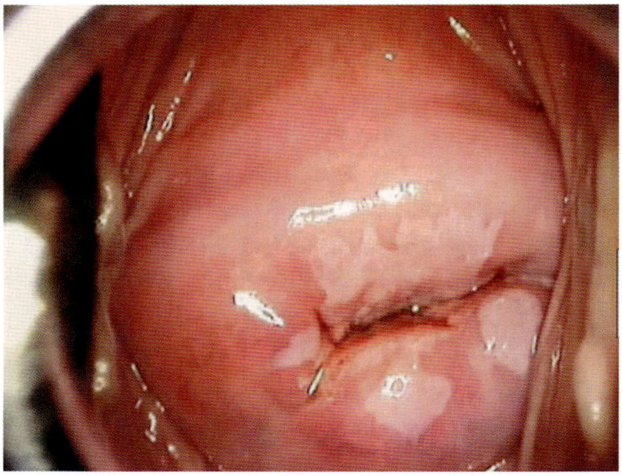

Fig. 17: After acidic acid for low-grade lesions.

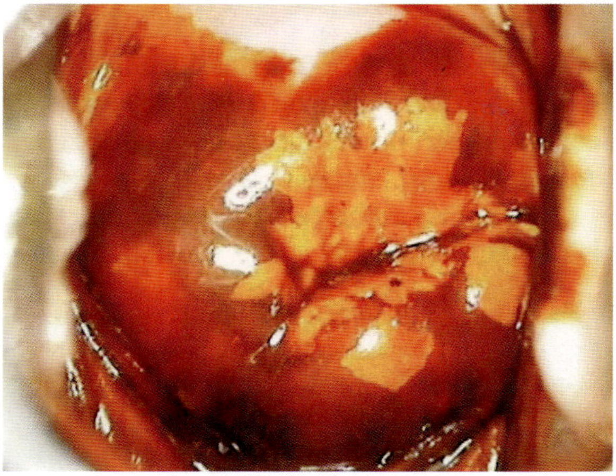

Fig. 18: After Lugol's iodine for low-grade lesions.

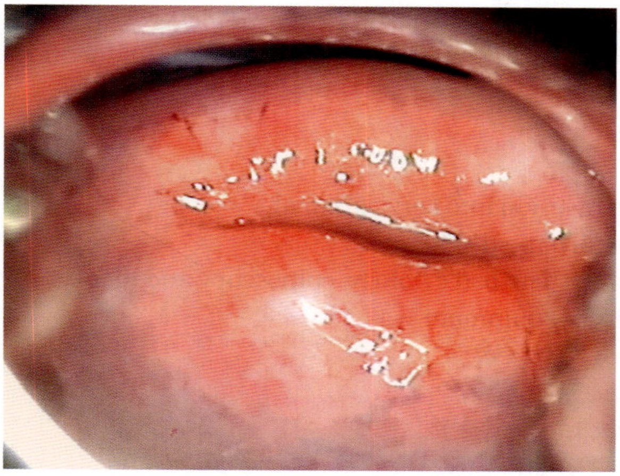

Fig. 19: After normal saline for high-grade lesions.

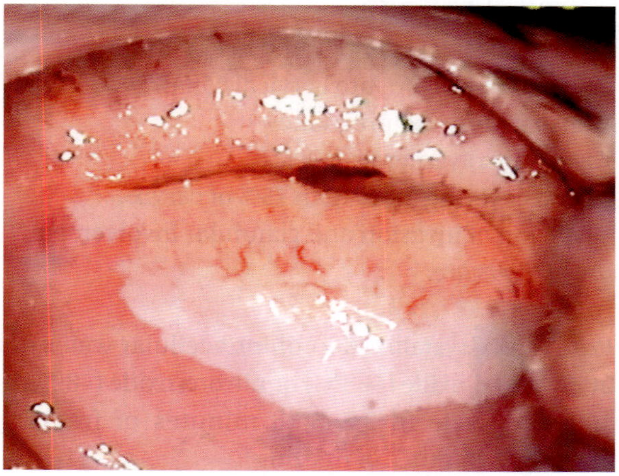

Fig. 20: After acidic acid for high-grade lesions.

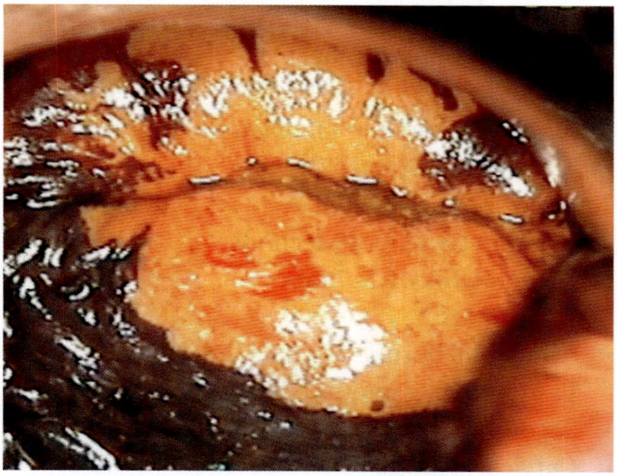

Fig. 21: After Lugol's iodine for high-grade lesions.

Factors determining the selection of treatment methods:

- Whether or not the woman has completed her childbearing
- Grade of lesion
- Size of lesion
- Type of TZ
- Extension of lesion into cervical canal
- Vaginal involvement
- Concordance between cytology, colposcopy and biopsy
- Availability of equipment

Methods of treatment:

I. *Ablative methods:*
    - *Indications:*
        - CIN1 and CIN2
        - Occasionally CIN3 in young women
    - *Contraindications:*
        - Type 2 and Type 3 TZ
        - Discordance bet cytology and histopathology
        - Extension of lesion into cervical canal
        - Menstruation and pregnancy
        - Vaginal involvement
        - Lesion covering more than 75% of cervix
        - Suspicion of invasion and glandular involvement

Ablative methods are:

1. *Cryotherapy:*
    - *Principal:* Crystallization of intracellular water due to freezing by carbon dioxide (–68°C) or nitrous oxide (–89°C).
    - *Method:* Cycle of 3-5-3 (3 minutes of freezing–5 minutes thawing–3 minutes of freezing)
    - *Complications:*
        - Pain
        - Vasomotor symptoms (rare)
        - Secondary hemorrhage
        - PID
2. *Cold coagulation or thermal ablation:*
    - *Indications:* CIN2 and CIN3
    - *Temperature:* 100–120°C
    - *Application time:* 20–45 seconds
    - *Depth of treatment:* 5–7 mm
    - *Complications:*
        - Accidental burn of vagina
        - Vasomotor symptoms (fainting, giddiness)
        - Secondary hemorrhage
        - Cervical stenosis

3. *LASER ablation/vaporization*: Due to expensive instruments and special training required to operate; LASER vaporization is a lesser used treatment of method.

II. *Excisional methods:*
- Loop Electrosurgical Excision Procedure (LEEP):
  - Colposcopic-guided biopsy
  - Done by Punch biopsy forces or LEEP electrode.
  - The smallest size of loop electrode is selected.
  - Biopsy site is infiltrated by 1% xylocaine solution.
  - Small CIN1 and CIN2 can be treated by LEEP.
- Large Loop Excision of Transformation Zone (LLETZ):

1. *Indications:*
   - Biopsy proven HSIL
   - TZ type 2 and 3
   - More than 75% cervix covered with lesion
   - Extension of lesion in cervical canal
   - Persistent lesion after ablative treatment
   - Discordance between cytology, colposcopy, and biopsy
2. *Complications:*
   - Excessive bleeding during and after procedure
   - Postoperative infections
   - Treatment failure in about 10% patients
   - Needle Excision of Transformation Zone (NETZ)
   - Straight Wire Excision of Transformation Zone (SWETZ)
   - Cold Knife Conization (CKC)
   - Laser conization

III. *Postoperative protocol for all procedures:*
- Oral antibiotics for 5 days
- Abstinence for 6–8 weeks
- Follow-up at 6 months.

SUGGESTED READING

1. Colposcopy Digital Atlas: Principles and Practice. International Agency for Research on Cancer
2. Principles and Practice of Colposcopy. 3rd Edition. B Shakuntala Baliga

19

CHAPTER

Fertility Preservation in Gynecological Cancer

Rohan Palshetkar, Nandita Palshetkar, Mayuri More, Chiranjeev Shetty

INTRODUCTION

Gynecologic cancers are very common among females, with an estimated global incidence of 222,700 novel cases in Europe.

In the last ten years, approximately 20% of patients have undergone their initial pregnancy after the age of 40, resulting in an increased likelihood of cancer development before achieving reproductive goals. A considerable percentage of patients diagnosed with gynecologic cancers are of reproductive age and have not realized their aspiration to establish a family.

Nevertheless, unlike other types of tumors, gonadotoxicity induced by medical and/or radiation therapy was not the primary reason which is responsible for infertility.

The gynecologic cancer diagnosis might impact fertility from an anatomical perspective, particularly when surgical intervention results in irreversible damage. The consideration of fertility preservation is a significant concern in this context.

Consequently, the majority of scientific information about fertility preservation in gynecologic cancers predominantly emphasizes surgical intervention.

RADIATION THERAPY

Radiation therapy targeting abdomen and pelvis is related to a considerable risk of permanent amenorrhea and may adversely affect the uterus as well as uterine arteries, compromising a woman's ability "to carry a pregnancy to term".

The probability of radiation sequelae rises with progressive disease stage, substantial residual tumor size, as well as abdominal carcinomatosis. Innovations in radiation approaches, like intensity-modulated radiation therapy (IMRT) as well as proton therapy, might permit radiotherapists to protect the ovaries as well as uterus from significant radiation exposure, consequently reducing possible detrimental impacts on fertility. Cerebral irradiation may potentially lead to amenorrhea and infertility.

Ovarian dysfunction: Abdominopelvic irradiation can directly impact on the gonads, resulting in sterility. A newborn girl possesses around 2 million oocytes within her ovaries, undergoing meiotic division, that concludes immediately prior to ovulation years subsequently.[12] The number of oocytes declines as the age increases until menopause, at which time only a finite quantity of oocytes remains viable.

Direct DNA damage to ovarian follicles can occur due to ionizing radiation, resulting in follicular atrophy and a consequent reduction in ovarian follicular reserve. Oocytes have considerable radiosensitivity.

Uterine dysfunction: Uterine irradiation may elevate the likelihood of complications during pregnancy, including spontaneous miscarriage, preterm labor as well as delivery, fetal malposition, premature low birth weight, as well as placental attachment abnormalities. RT-related uterine dysfunctions mostly stem from myometrial fibrosis, vascular impairment of the uterus, and endometrial destruction. Damage to the uterine vasculature might lead to inadequate vascularization and, as a result, diminished feto-placental blood flow, restricting fetal growth. Placental abnormalities are associated with endometrial injury and the suppression of normal decidualization.

Hypothalamic-pituitary-ovarian axis dysfunction: Dysfunction of the hypothalamic–pituitary–ovarian axis is an identified possible secondary consequence of cranial irradiation. The development of endocrinopathy is dependent on damage to the hypothalamus and/or pituitary gland caused by radiation therapy. The hypothalamic–pituitary–ovarian axis governs menstruation and fertility via the release of follicle-stimulating hormone (FSH), prolactin, luteinizing hormone (LH), estradiol, progesterone, and gonadotropin-releasing hormone (GnRH). Nonetheless, this potential outcome holds minimal relevance for most gynecologic patients who do not exhibit brain metastases at the time of diagnosis.

CHEMOTHERAPY

The impact of chemotherapeutic medicines on ovarian function markedly differs with age, as demonstrated in other cancers, and is affected by the chemotherapy protocol, comprising type, dosage, number of cycles, and medication mechanism of action. The primary chemotherapeutic agents employed in gynecological oncology comprise alkylating agents such as cyclophosphamide as well as ifosfamide, platinum compounds including cisplatin as well as carboplatin, taxanes like paclitaxel, anthracyclines such as doxorubicin, and antimetabolites including gemcitabine and 5-fluorouracil **(Table 1)**.

TABLE 1: Chemotherapy agents used in gynecological cancer.

Drugs	*Mechanism of action*	*Target cell*	*Risk of amenorrhea*
Alkylating agents • Cyclophosphamide • Ifosfamide	Single-stranded DNA breaks	• Non primordial follicles • Primordial follicles • Follicular atresia	High
Platinums • Cisplatin • Carboplatin	Inter- and intra-strand DNA cross-links; chromosomal damage	Oocyte	Intermediate
Taxanes Paclitaxel	Inhibition of microtubule formation and spindle functions	• Primordial follicles • Granulosa cells	Intermediate
Anthracyclines Doxorubicin	Inhibition of DNA replication and transcription	• Stromal tissue • Granulosa cells	Low
Antimetabolites • Gemcitabine • 5-fluorouracil	Alteration DNA synthesis	• Pre-antral • Antral	Low

Alkylating compounds are chemotherapeutic substances that demonstrate gonadotoxic effects, which are consistently related to ovarian failure in a dose-dependent way. Alkylating chemicals cause damage to oocytes through single-stranded DNA degrades and impact cells at all phases of the cell cycle, particularly targeting primordial follicles.[18] The effect of taxanes as well as platinum on fertility poses a moderate risk (30–70%) for amenorrhea, but treatment protocols that include antimetabolites and anthracyclines have been associated with a reduced risk (below 30%).[4] The inclusion of anthracyclines in taxane-based regimens appears to increase levels of gonadotoxicity.

FERTILITY PRESERVATION STRATEGIES

Strategies for fertility preservation are predominantly determined by patient attributes, including age and the choice between utilizing male partner or donor sperm, alongside tumor attributes such as disease stage, histology, and treatment alternatives. Oncofertility counseling is important for advising cancer patients about the dangers of treatment-induced premature ovarian failure as well as infertility linked to certain anticancer therapies. It also outlines several alternatives for maintaining ovarian function and fertility, providing an analysis of the benefits and drawbacks of each option.

Table 2 represents a summary of the primary techniques for fertility preservation. **Flowchart 1** represents fertility preservation techniques corresponding to each type of gynecological cancer, supplementing the information in **Table 2**.

Flowchart 1: Fertility preservation techniques corresponding to each type of gynecological cancer.

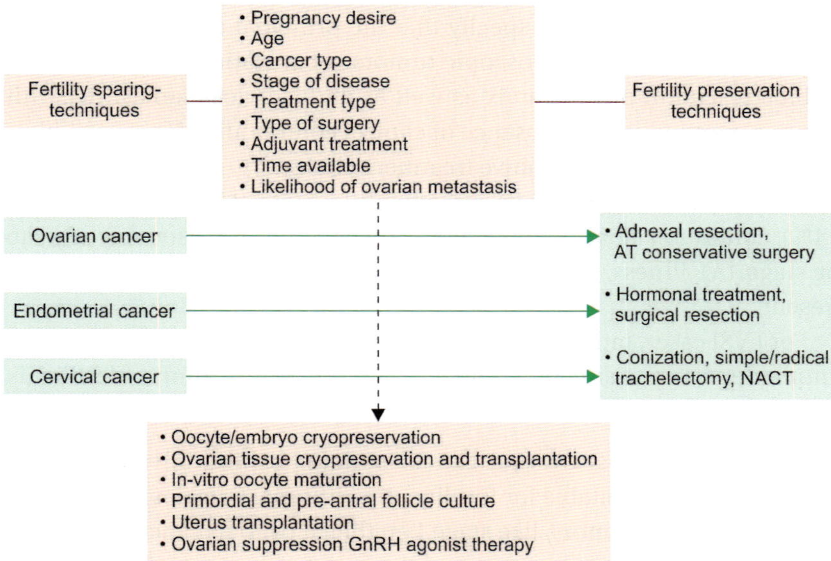

TABLE 2: Primary techniques for fertility preservation.

Strategy	*Definition*
Surgical option	
Conization	Removal of the ectocervix and endocervical canals
Radical trachelectomy	Removal of the cervix with preservation of the uterus
Ovarian transposition	Transposition of ovaries out of the radiation field
Unilateral oophorectomy	Removal of one ovary
Medical option	
Progestin-based therapy	Progestin therapy and endometrial curettage
GnRHa	GnRHa-based therapy
Assisted option	
Embryo cryopreservation	In vitro fertilization of oocytes, then cryopreserved
Oocyte cryopreservation	Unfertilized oocyte cryopreservation
Ovarian cryopreservation	Removal of ovarian tissue, then cryopreserved

SURGICAL AND MEDICAL OPTIONS

Cervical cancer: The approach to cervical cancer management must be modified according to the disease's individual stage. Conization along with trachelectomy is often suggested for early-stage cervical cancer (stage IA–IB1). The conventional treatment for later stages (stage >IB1) is radiotherapy, with or without chemotherapy. Nonetheless, neoadjuvant chemotherapy succeeded by major surgery is regarded as a feasible alternative.

International protocols specify that the principal diagnostic as well as treatment strategy for microscopic tumors is conization, that involves the en bloc resection of ectocervix as well as endocervical canals. Regarding negative margins and the absence of clinical contraindications, cone biopsy might be regarded as a definitive treatment choice.

Furthermore, because of its exceedingly low rate of lymphatic metastasis (<1%), conization alone, without lymphadenectomy, is reasonably advisable for stage IA1 illness, when lymphovascular space invasion (LVSI) is not present.

For LVSI cases, radical trachelectomy combined with laparoscopic pelvic lymphadenectomy is recommended when the preservation of fertility is a priority.

Ovarian cancer: Most ovarian cancer patients exhibit advanced illness, rendering them unsuitable for fertility preservation strategies. Borderline as well as early-stage tumors, like stage I epithelial ovarian cancers, malignant ovarian germ cell tumors, and sex cord stromal tumors may be appropriate candidates for fertility-preserving surgical techniques. However, although recurrence after conservative treatment, even in IA stage, is a realistic instance, many authors support the application of adjuvant platinum-based chemotherapy in order to reduce present risk.

Endometrial cancer: It primarily impacts postmenopausal women. Endometrial cancer in reproductive-age women often has a clinical history of polycystic ovarian syndrome, it lowers the possibility of conception and must be regarded when prescribing fertility-sparing treatment. Patients having stage IA illness seeking to fertility preservation may be recommended a fertility-sparing strategy. Continuous progestin medication, followed by numerous endometrial curettages, is suitable for low-risk, well-differentiated endometrioid carcinoma. Most research on this subject suggests that the duration of treatment must be on the basis of treatment response after a minimum of 3 months; individuals displaying chronic or worsening disease after 6–9 months must be assessed for radical surgery. Fertility preservation is contraindicated in cases "of serous carcinoma, clear cell carcinoma, or carcinosarcoma histology. If fertility preservation" has been selected, a hysterectomy is advised following deliveries.

ASSISTED REPRODUCTIVE ALTERNATIVES

The conventional methods for maintaining assisted reproduction involve cryopreservation of embryos and oocytes. Cryopreservation should be conducted prior to the initiation of cancer treatment to provide the chance to preserve fertility.

Embryo cryopreservation: The most recognized approach for fertility preservation is employed when the patient does not necessitate the early commencement of cancer therapy. It requires donor sperm or a male partner. Embryo cryopreservation is a reliable approach. The procedure involves random ovarian stimulation with the administration of gonadotropins for a duration of 8–14 days, or initiating treatment within 3 days following the commencement "of the menstrual cycle. Subsequent to retrieval, oocytes are assessed for maturity, fertilized, and subsequently cryopreserved.

Oocyte cryopreservation: The process of cryopreservation of unfertilized oocytes needs ovarian stimulation by daily gonadotropin injections as well as ultrasound-guided oocyte retrieval completed under anesthesia. This approach is specifically significant for patients without a male partner or those choosing not to utilize donor sperm. Oocyte freezing is related to lower conception rates compared to embryo cryopreservation.

Ovarian cryopreservation: The cryopreservation of ovarian tissue is presently regarded as an experimental method for preserving reproductive potential. The ovarian cortex contains a significant concentration of inactive primordial follicles, with oocytes arrested in the diplotene phase of the first meiotic prophase. The ideal candidates for this operation are women under forty, because of their increased ovarian reserve. A companion is not required, and ovarian stimulation is unnecessary, leading to no postponement at the start of treatment. Cortical ovarian tissue, measuring between 0.5 and 2 cm, is obtained using laparoscopy and cryopreserved for possible reimplantation or in vitro egg maturation.

ALTERNATIVE STRATEGIES

Gonadotropin-releasing hormone agonists (GnRHa) represent an experimental strategy aimed to suppress ovarian function during chemotherapy (CHT). In theory, GnRHa administration diminishes gonadotropin levels, inducing an artificial prepubertal condition in the ovaries. Furthermore, investigations of ovarian tissue have resulted in the idea that these chemicals may mitigate organ damage and local ischemia induced by chemotherapy drugs. Administration should ideally commence 2–4 weeks prior to chemotherapy. Recent investigations demonstrate that GnRHa might have a protective function in prolonging the onset of early menopause while facilitating a favorable pregnancy rate. GnRHa has been associated with menopausal-like symptoms, that include hot flashes, headaches, decreased bone density, sweating, and mood changes.

Their application has been extensively studied regarding fertility preservation for breast cancer patients, although less data exists regarding their utilization in gynecologic malignancies.

Nevertheless, a potential role for fertility preservation in gynecologic cancers may be suggested to reduce ovarian failure that may occur after conservative surgical treatment for ovarian cancer or to implement neoadjuvant strategies before conservative surgeries for early-stage cervical tumors.

Current and prospective outlooks for women who have undergone hysterectomy (excluding uterine transplantation): All the treatments mentioned thus far may be relevant for early-stage cancers that do not require the excision "of reproductive organs. The exclusive options for women who have undergone hysterectomy to attain motherhood are legal adoption" or gestational surrogacy following oocyte or embryo preservation.

Uterus transplantation that occurs "in benign and malignant conditions necessitates immunosuppressive agents' high doses, poses a risk of cancer recurrence in patients with" immune systems that are compromised, and presents a probability of vascular abnormalities post-pelvic radiation, thereby requiring meticulous assessment before seeking this option for cancer patients.

Nevertheless, it may represent an innovative approach for handling gynecologic cancer patients seeking fertility preservation.

FERTILITY ISSUES WITH BRCA CARRIERS

Women possessing germline mutations in *BRCA* genes have a markedly increased lifelong risk of ovarian cancer as well as breast cancer. To reduce cancer risk and improve survival, risk-reduction procedures must be performed at the age of 25. Though women with BRCA mutations are more likely than those without to develop breast cancer earlier in life, choices about risk-reducing salpingo-oophorectomy (RRSO) and bilateral risk-reducing mastectomy (BRRM) need to be made after a comprehensive, evidence-based analysis of the benefits and drawbacks of preventive surgery. RRSO is advised for BRCA mutation carriers to mitigate the risk of ovarian and fallopian tube cancer by the age of 40 or following the conclusion of childbearing. This preventive method involves considerable restrictions on reproductive capacity and may offer health hazards associated with early menopause.

Moreover, there is disagreement regarding the fertility potential in this patient population. BRCA germline mutations appear to correlate with diminished ovarian reserve, resulting in a reduced reproductive lifetime relative to women who do not have BRCA mutations. The dysfunction of BRCA predisposes individuals to DNA damage, resulting in heightened follicular atresia and apoptotic oocytes. Presently, early fertility counseling has been advised.

CONCLUSION

The actual efficacy of various treatments for fertility preservation in gynecologic malignancies requires assessment. The primary reason for infertility is the surgical removal of reproductive organs; thus, altering the surgical procedure is the most advisable course of action.

Embryo and oocyte cryopreservation are recognized as conventional treatments and are readily accessible for many tumors; these techniques may also be employed in gynecologic cancers, particularly in scenarios requiring uterus-sparing or uterus-surrogate carriers. Alternative fertility preservation techniques must be considered experimental and designated for individuals undergoing therapy at specialized centers with the necessary expertise.

Patients as well as clinicians must prioritize cancer diagnosis; nonetheless, the patient and her family must get thorough counseling on fertility preservation. The dangers associated with conservative therapy must be evaluated in relation to the drawbacks of more aggressive treatment alternatives. The patient must understand that opting for fertility-sparing treatment entails a lesser, but ambiguous, chance of disease recurrence. Nevertheless, patients and professionals must assess the realistic probability of conception on the basis of the patient's age, family history, and fertility evaluation.

It is essential that a multidisciplinary team review, comprising gynecologic oncologists, radiation oncologists, medical oncologists, reproductive endocrinologists, and perinatologists, becomes standard practice. Thus, the engagement of a psychologist is essential for providing precise details to patients suffering from gynecological cancer who seek to maintain their reproductive capacity.

SUGGESTED READING

1. Bastings L, Baysal Ö, Beerendonk CC, et al. Deciding about fertility preservation after specialist counselling. Hum Reprod. 2014;29(8):1721-9. https://doi.org/10.1093/humrep/deu136 PMID: 24916435.
2. Brännström M, Diaz-Garcia C, Johannesson L, et al. Livebirth after uterus transplantation. Lancet. 2015:385(9968);607-16. https://doi.org/10.1016/S0140-6736(14)61728-1.
3. Brearley SG, Stamataki Z, Addington-Hall J, et al. The physical and practical problems experienced by cancer survivors: a rapid review and synthesis of the literature. Eur J Oncol Nurs. 2011;15(3):204-12. https://doi.org/10.1016/j.ejon.2011.02.005 PMID: 21489873.

4. Chan JL, Wang ET. Oncofertility for women with gynecologic malignancies. Gynecol Oncol. 2016;144(3):631-6. https://doi.org/10.1016/j.ygyno.2016.12.013 PMID: 28012689.
5. Chiarelli AM, Marrett LD, Darlington GA, et al. Pregnancy outcomes in females after treatment for childhood cancer. Epidemiology. 2000;11(2): 161-6. https://doi.org/10.1097/00001648-20000300000013 PMID: 11021613.
6. De Felice F, Marchetti C, Musella A, et al. Bilateral risk-reduction mastectomy in BRCA1 and BRCA2 mutation carriers: a meta-analysis. Ann Surg Oncol. 2015;22(9):2876-80. https://doi.org/10.1245/s10434-015-4532-1 PMID: 25808098.
7. De Felice F, Marchetti C. Risk-reducing surgery in BRCA1/2 mutation carries: a point of view. Oncotarget. 2015;6(37):39391-2. https://doi.org/10.18632/oncotarget.6348 PMID: 26588056 PMCID: 4741830.
8. de la Noval BD. Potential implications on female fertility and reproductive lifespan in BRCA germline mutation women. Arch Gynecol Obstet. 2016;294(5): 1099-103. https://doi.org/10.1007/s00404-016-4187-6 PMID:27561295.
9. Elgindy E, Sibai H, Abdelghani A, et al. Protecting ovaries during chemotherapy through gonad suppression: a systematic review and meta-analysis. Obstet Gynecol. 2015;126(1):187-95. https://doi.org/10.1097/AOG.0000000000000905 PMID: 26241272.
10. Ferlay J, Steliarova-Foucher E, Lortet-Tieulent J, et al. Cancer incidence and mortality patterns in Europe: estimates for 40 countries in 2012. Eur J Cancer. 2013;49(6):1374-403. https://doi.org/10.1016/j.ejca.2012.12.027 PMID: 23485231.
11. Finer LB, Philbin JM. Trends in ages at key reproductive transitions in the United States, 1951–2010. Womens Health Issues. 2014;e271–e279. https://doi.org/10.1016/j.whi.2014.02.002.
12. Gracia CR, Sammel MD, and Freeman E, et al. Impact of cancer therapies on ovarian reserve. Fertil Steril. 2012;97(1):134-40. https://doi.org/10.1016/j.fertnstert.2011.10.040.
13. Hickman LC, Valentine LN, Falcone T, et al. Preservation of gonadal function in women undergoing chemotherapy: a review of the potential role for gonadotropin-releasing hormone agonists. Am J Obstet Gynecol. 2016;215(4):415-22. https://doi.org/10.1016/j.ajog.2016.06.053 PMID: 27422055.
14. Kvarnström N, Järvholm S, Johannesson L, et al. Live donors of the initial observational study of uterus transplantation-psychological and medical follow-up until 1 year after surgery in the 9 cases. Transplantation. 2017;101(3):664-70. https://doi.org/10.1097/TP.0000000000001567.
15. Laganà AS, La Rosa VL, Rapisarda AM, et al. Comment on "Needs and priorities of women with endometrial and cervical cancer". J Psychosom Obstet Gynaecol. 2015;38(1):85-6. https://doi.org/10.1080/0167482X.2016.1244186.
16. Landoni F, Parma G, Peiretti M, et al. Chemo-conization in early cervical cancer. Gynecol Oncol. 2007;107(1 Suppl 1):S125-6. https://doi.org/10.1016/j.ygyno.2007.07.011 PMID: 17727935.
17. Larsen EC, Schmiegelow K, Rechnitzer C, et al. Radiotherapy at a young age reduces uterine volume of childhood cancer survivors. Acta Obstet Gynecol Scand. 2004;83(1):96-102. https://doi.org/10.1111/j.1600-0412.2004.00332.x.

18. Lawson AK, Klock SC, Pavone ME, et al. Psychological counseling of female fertility preservation patients. J Psychosoc Oncol. 2015;33(4):333-53.https://doi.org/10.1080/07347332.2015.1045677 PMID: 25996581 PMCID: 4557874.
19. Levine JM, Kelvin JF, Quinn GP, et al. Infertility in reproductive-age female cancer survivors. Cancer. 2015;121(10):1532-9. https://doi.org/10.1002/cncr.29181 PMID: 25649243.
20. Loren AW, Mangu PB, Beck LN, et al. Fertility preservation for patients with cancer: American Society of Clinical Oncology Clinical Practice Guideline Update. J Clin Oncol. 2013;31(19):2500-10. https://doi.org/10.1200/JCO.2013.49.2678. PMID: 23715580 PMCID:5321083.
21. Marchetti C, De Felice F, Palaia I, et al. Risk-reducing salpingo-oophorectomy: a meta-analysis on impact on ovarian cancer risk and all-cause mortality in BRCA1 and BRCA2 mutation carriers. BMC Womens Health. 2014;14:150. https://doi.org/10.1186/s12905-014-0150-5 PMID: 25494812 PMCID:4271468.
22. Marchetti C, Iadarola R, Palaia I, et al. Hormone therapy in oophorectomized BRCA1/2 mutation carriers. Menopause. 2014;21(7):763-8. https://doi.org/10.1097/GME.0000000000000126.
23. McCorkle R, Tang ST, Greenwald H, et al. Factors related to depressive symptoms among long-term survivors of cervical cancer. Health Care Women Int. 2006;27(1):45-58. https://doi.org/10.1080/07399330500377507.
24. Munhoz RR, Pereira AA, Sasse AD, et al. Gonadotropin-releasing hormone agonists for ovarian function preservation in premenopausal women undergoing chemotherapy for early-stage breast cancer: a systematic review and meta-analysis. JAMA Oncol. 2016;2(1):65-73. https://doi.org/10.1001/jamaoncol.2015.3251 PMCID: 5003018.
25. National Comprehensive Cancer Network [http://www.nccn.org] Date Accessed: 19/01/17.
26. Ogilvy-Stuart AL and Shalet SM. Effect of radiation on the human reproductive system. Environ Health Perspect. 1993;101(Suppl 2):109-16. https://doi.org/10.1289/ehp.93101s2109 PMID: 8243379 PMCID: 1519954.
27. Oktem O, Urman B. Options of fertility preservation in female cancer patients. Obstet Gynecol Surv. 2010;65(8):531-42. https://doi.org/10.1097/OGX.0b013e3181f8c0aa PMID: 20955632.
28. Ozyurt BE, et al. A descriptive study about social support perceived by cancer patients. Kriz Dergisi (Journal of Crisis). 2007;15:1-15.
29. Pfeifer S, Goldberg J, Lobo R, et al. Ovarian tissue cryopreservation: a committee opinion. Fertil Steril. 2014;101(5):1237-43. https://doi.org/10.1016/j.fertnstert.2014.02.052.
30. Rockall AG, Qureshi MI, Papadopoulou I, et al. Role of imaging in fertility-sparing treatment of gynecologic malignancies. Radiographics. 2016;36(7):2214-33. https://doi.org/10.1148/rg.2016150254 PMID: 27831834.
31. Rosen R, Brown C, Heiman J, et al. The Female Sexual Function Index (FSFI): a multidimensional self-report instrument for the assessment of female sexual function. J Sex Marital Ther. 2000;26(2):191-208. https://doi.org/10.1080/009262300278597 PMID: 10782451.
32. Sella T, Mironov S, Hricak H. Imaging of transposed ovaries in patients with cervical carcinoma. Am J Roentgenol. 2005;184(5):1602-10. https://doi.org/10.2214/ajr.184.5.01841602 PMID: 15855125.

33. Taylor JF, Rosen RC, Leiblum SR. Self-report assessment of female sexual function: psychometric evaluation of the Brief Index of Sexual Functioning for Women. Arch Sex Behav. 1994;23(6):627-43. https://doi.org/10.1007/BF01541816 PMID: 7872859.
34. Tomao F, Corrado G, Peccatori FA, et al. Fertility-sparing options in young women with cervical cancer. Curr Treat Options Oncol. 2016;17(1): 5. https://doi.org/10.1007/s11864-015-0386-9 PMID: 26810054.
35. Tomao F, Maruccio M, Preti EP, et al. Conization in early stage cervical cancer: pattern of recurrence in a 10-year single-institution experience. Int J Gynecol Cancer. 2017;27(5):1001-8. https://doi.org/10.1097/IGC.0000000000000991 PMID: 28486242.
36. Tomao F, Peccatori F, Del Pup L, et al. Special issues in fertility preservation for gynecologic malignancies. Crit Rev Oncol Hematol.2016;97:206-19. https://doi.org/10.1016/j.critrevonc.2015.08.024.
37. Vitale SG La Rosa VL, Rapisarda AM, et al. Comment on "Anxiety and depression in patients with advanced ovarian cancer: a prospective study". Psychosom Obstet Gynaecol. 2017;38(1):83-4. https://doi.org/10.1080/0167482X.2016.1244182.
38. Vitale SG La Rosa VL, Rapisarda AM, et al. Comment on "The consequences of gynaecological cancer in patients and their partners from the sexual and psychological perspective". J Cancer Res Ther. 2017;13(3): 598-9 PMID:28862236.
39. Vitale SG, La Rosa VL, Rapisarda AM, et al. Psychology of infertility and assisted reproductive treatment: the Italian situation. J Psychosom Obstet Gynecol.2017;38(1):1-3. https://doi.org/10.1080/0167482X.2016.1244184.
40. Vitale SG, La Rosa VL, Rapisarda AM, et al. Psychology of infertility and assisted reproductive treatment: the Italian situation. J Psychosom Obstet Gynecol. 2017;38(1):1-3. https://doi.org/10.1080/0167482X.2016.1244184.
41. Vitale SG, La Rosa VL, Rapisarda AMC, et al. The importance of fertility preservation counseling in patients with gynecologic cancer. J Reprod Infertil. 2017;18(2);261-3. PMID: 28868252 PMCID: 5565906.
42. Vitale SG, Petrosino B, La Rosa VL, et al. Comment on "Differences in psychophysical well-being and signs of depression in couples undergoing their first consultation for assisted reproduction technology (ART): an Italian pilot study." Eur J Obstet Gynecol Reprod Biol. 2016;211:210-11. https://doi.org/10.1016/j.ejogrb.2016.10.029.
43. Wallace WH, Thomson AB, Saran F, et al. Predicting age of ovarian failure after radiation to a field that includes the ovaries. Int J Radiat Oncol Biol Phys. 2005;62(3):738-44. https://doi.org/10.1016/j.ijrobp.2004.11.038 PMID: 15936554.
44. Wenzel LB, Donnelly JP, Fowler JM, et al. Resilience, reflection, and residual stress in ovarian cancer survivorship: a gynecologic oncology group study. Psychooncology. 2002;11(2):142-53. https://doi.org/10.1002/pon.567 PMID: 11921330.
45. Wo JY, Viswanathan AN. Impact of radiotherapy on fertility, pregnancy, and neonatal outcomes in female cancer patients. Int J Radiat Oncol Biol Phys. 2009;73(5):1304-12. https://doi.org/10.1016/j.ijrobp.2008.12.016 PMID: 19306747 PMCID:2865903.